SpringerBriefs in Modern Perspectives on Disability Research

Series Editors

Gabriel Bennett, Independent Researcher, Klemzig, Australia

Emma Goodall, Healthy Possibilities, Seaford, Australia

This book series on disability research is a comprehensive collection of research on disability and related issues. The series is designed to promote interdisciplinary collaboration and exchange, bringing together scholars and practitioners from different fields to share their perspectives and insights. Disability research is an interdisciplinary field that examines the social, cultural, historical, and political dimensions of disability. It encompasses a wide range of topics, including disability rights, accessibility, assistive technologies, healthcare, education, employment, and social welfare. Disability research scholars employ a range of theoretical and methodological approaches to understand the experiences of people with disabilities, as well as the ways in which disability intersects with other social identities such as race, gender, sexuality, and class.

The series seeks to advance knowledge and understanding of disability by publishing rigorous, innovative, and relevant research. It aims to promote disability rights and social justice by highlighting the ways in which people with disabilities are marginalized and discriminated against in society, and advocating for greater social inclusion and accessibility. The series also seeks to inform policy and practice by disseminating research findings that can help to shape policy decisions and contribute to positive social change.

Rishabha Malviya · Shivam Rajput

Advances and Insights into AI-Created Disability Supports

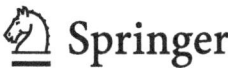
Springer

Rishabha Malviya
Department of Pharmacy, School
of Medical and Allied Sciences
Galgotias University
Greater Noida, Uttar Pradesh, India

Shivam Rajput
Department of Pharmacy, School
of Medical and Allied Sciences
Galgotias University
Greater Noida, Uttar Pradesh, India

ISSN 3004-9709　　　　　　　　ISSN 3004-9717　(electronic)
SpringerBriefs in Modern Perspectives on Disability Research
ISBN 978-981-96-6068-1　　　ISBN 978-981-96-6069-8　(eBook)
https://doi.org/10.1007/978-981-96-6069-8

© The Editor(s) (if applicable) and The Author(s), under exclusive license to Springer Nature Singapore Pte Ltd. 2025

This work is subject to copyright. All rights are solely and exclusively licensed by the Publisher, whether the whole or part of the material is concerned, specifically the rights of translation, reprinting, reuse of illustrations, recitation, broadcasting, reproduction on microfilms or in any other physical way, and transmission or information storage and retrieval, electronic adaptation, computer software, or by similar or dissimilar methodology now known or hereafter developed.

The use of general descriptive names, registered names, trademarks, service marks, etc. in this publication does not imply, even in the absence of a specific statement, that such names are exempt from the relevant protective laws and regulations and therefore free for general use.

The publisher, the authors and the editors are safe to assume that the advice and information in this book are believed to be true and accurate at the date of publication. Neither the publisher nor the authors or the editors give a warranty, expressed or implied, with respect to the material contained herein or for any errors or omissions that may have been made. The publisher remains neutral with regard to jurisdictional claims in published maps and institutional affiliations.

This Springer imprint is published by the registered company Springer Nature Singapore Pte Ltd.
The registered company address is: 152 Beach Road, #21-01/04 Gateway East, Singapore 189721, Singapore

If disposing of this product, please recycle the paper.

Foreword

The book *Advances and Insights into Artificial Intelligence Created Disability Supports* explores the role of AI in transforming the lives of disabled persons, breaking barriers, and inclusivity in disability support. The book, authored by Dr. Rishabha Malviya, is an indicator of optimism and possibility that goes beyond scholarly investigation. The book follows the evolution of artificial intelligence in disability care, from its historical beginnings to current breakthroughs and future possibilities. It discusses AI-powered assistive devices, personalized support using generative models, and innovations that improve communication and autonomy. The variety of issues covered, combined with real-world applications and critical observations, makes this book an excellent resource.

The authors emphasize the role of ethical considerations and inclusive design in AI's ability to uplift, empower, and create a more accessible society. As AI evolves, it is our common obligation to ensure that technical developments are used to break down systemic obstacles and promote equity for everyone. The book believes that Advances and Insights into Artificial Intelligence Created Disability Supports will stimulate innovation, spark significant conversations, and serve as a foundation for future study in this critical area. I express heartfelt gratitude to Dr. Rishabha Malviya and Shivam Rajput for their persistent efforts and dedication to compile a book that goals to develop a future in which technology supports humanity's ideal goals.

Happy Reading & Best Wishes

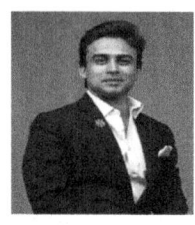

Dr. Dhruv Galgotia
CEO
Galgotias University
Greater Noida, India

Preface

The book *Advances and Insights into Artificial Intelligence Created Disability Supports* is a comprehensive discussion of the integration of AI into disability support systems. The book highlights the persistent difficulties that persons with disabilities face in everyday life, such as communication, transport, education, and healthcare. AI has started to overcome these gaps by providing innovative remedies that are tailored to individual needs, promote autonomy, and improve quality of life.

The book has been lined up to give readers a thorough overview of the development, recent breakthroughs, and potential applications of AI-driven disability care. It offers background information, demonstrates innovative developments, and looks ahead to the next phase of widely available technology.

The initial chapters describe the fundamental function of AI in disability support and its historical growth, emphasizing the possible progress of AI research with adaptive technology. The subsequent chapters explore the practical applications of AI, demonstrating the role of machine learning, natural language processing, and generative AI to customize, personalize, and improve support systems.

The book focuses on the human factor of AI in disability support, emphasizing the significance of inclusive design, ethical considerations, and ongoing engagement with the disability community. The future of AI in disability support is limitless, but its success is dependent on our collective willingness to use technology as a tool of empowerment rather than exclusion.

The book *Advances and Insights into Artificial Intelligence Created Disability Supports* intends to educate and inspire readers to consider and become involved in a future in which artificial intelligence is a fundamental component of human well-being and equality.

Greater Noida, India Rishabha Malviya
 Shivam Rajput

About This Book

The book "Advances and Insights into Artificial Intelligence Created Disability Supports" is an in-depth resource that explores the revolutionary potential of artificial intelligence (AI) in empowering persons with disabilities. The book explores the fundamental concepts of AI, its application in disability support, and its history, from early speech synthesis tools to modern AI-powered prosthetics and mobility aids. It highlights the societal benefits of AI-powered support systems, which promote independence and improve quality of life.

The book provides insight into the history of the impact of AI on disability support, documenting key breakthroughs from early speech synthesis tools to modern AI-powered prostheses and mobility aids. It focuses on practical instances of AI empowering people with disabilities, like voice-activated virtual assistants and AI-powered navigation devices for people with visual impairments.

The book additionally investigates AI-powered advances in assistive technology for persons with disabilities, such as smart wheelchairs, wearable health monitoring, and adaptive learning platforms. Generative AI advances boundaries in personalized support by adapting solutions to specific needs. It can develop customized educational materials, adaptable interfaces, and personalized rehabilitation programs, all of which improve user experience and support effectiveness.

With a focus on developments like real-time translation, speech-to-text apps, and emotion recognition software, the book additionally discusses the potential of AI to close communication gaps. It continues with a discussion of upcoming technologies, ethical issues, the significance of inclusive design, and an outline of the future of AI-driven disability care. The book promotes continued collaboration among engineers, healthcare practitioners, and disabled populations to ensure that AI evolves as a technology of empowerment.

Contents

1 **Introduction to the Role of Artificial Intelligence in Disability Support** 1
   1.1 Introduction 1
   1.2 Disabled Person Assistance with AI 3
   1.3 AI-Based Computer Vision for Assistive Technology Tasks 3
      1.3.1 Object Recognition 3
      1.3.2 Facial Recognition 5
      1.3.3 Gaze Detection 5
   1.4 Additional AI Assistive Technology 6
      1.4.1 Speech Recognition 6
      1.4.2 Facilitating Communication 7
      1.4.3 Vision Technology for Mobility Independence 8
      1.4.4 Autonomous Vehicles 8
      1.4.5 Autonomy-Promoting Cognitive Support 9
      1.4.6 Localization 10
   1.5 New Developments in Healthcare 11
      1.5.1 Precision Diagnosis 12
      1.5.2 Personalized Treatment Plans 12
      1.5.3 Rehabilitation and Prosthetics 13
   1.6 Inclusive Education 14
      1.6.1 Learning Opportunities 15
      1.6.2 Pathways to Personalized Education 16
      1.6.3 Revolutionizing Communication and Interaction 17
   1.7 AI Promoting Disabled Independence 18
   1.8 Conclusion 19
   References 19

2 **The History of AI in Transforming Disability Support** 25
   2.1 Introduction 25
   2.2 Introduction to Technology 27
   2.3 The Evolution of Assistive Devices 28

		2.3.1 The Foundation Period (Before 1900)	28
		2.3.2 The Establishment Period (1900–1972)	28
		2.3.3 The Empowerment Period (After 1973–Present)	29
	2.4	Evolution of Assistive Devices	30
		2.4.1 Ancient Roots of Assistive Technology	30
		2.4.2 Communication Advancement by Braille	31
		2.4.3 Evolution of Hearing Aids	32
		2.4.4 From Wheelchairs to Advanced Mobility Aids	33
		2.4.5 Communication by Computer Accessibility	34
		2.4.6 Smart Modern Innovative Devices	34
	2.5	The Future of Assistive Technology	36
		2.5.1 AI Enhancing Accessibility by Assistive Technology	36
		2.5.2 Daily Living Assistance	37
		2.5.3 BCI Techniques Advancing Assistive Technologies	38
	2.6	Conclusion	38
		References	39
3	**Empowering Disabled People with AI**		**43**
	3.1	Introduction	43
	3.2	AI Benefits for Disability Support	44
		3.2.1 Communication	44
		3.2.2 Assistance for the Visually Impaired	46
		3.2.3 Assistance for Deaf People	46
		3.2.4 Assistance for Physically Disabled	47
	3.3	Conversational Systems for Cognitive Disabilities	48
	3.4	Inclusive Design in Conversational AI	49
	3.5	Advanced Robotics for Physical Assistance	50
	3.6	Smart Wheelchair Mobility	50
	3.7	Smart Technologies for Rehabilitation and Exercise	51
	3.8	Assistance in Education for Disabled Students	52
	3.9	Empower Independent Living	53
	3.10	Equal Access to Services	54
	3.11	Conclusion	56
		References	56
4	**AI-Driven Innovations in Assistive Technology for People with Disabilities**		**61**
	4.1	Introduction	61
	4.2	Assistive Technologies	63
	4.3	AI-Based Assistive Technologies	63
		4.3.1 Voice Recognition	64
		4.3.2 Augmentative and Alternative Communication	65

		4.3.3 Speech Recognition and Natural Language Processing (NLP)	66
	4.4	AI-Based Computer Vision for Object Recognition	67
	4.5	AI-Enabled Prostheses Control	68
	4.6	AI-Enabled Exoskeletons	69
	4.7	AI-Enabled Wheelchairs	70
	4.8	Advanced Assistance by AI Through Human–Computer Interaction	72
	4.9	Conclusion	73
	References		74
5	**Personalized Support for People with Disabilities Through Generative AI**		79
	5.1	Introduction	79
	5.2	AI in Assistive Technology	80
	5.3	Application of AI for Personalized Support to Disabled	83
		5.3.1 Motion Detection for Enhanced Accessibility	83
		5.3.2 Visual Analysis for Accessibility	84
	5.4	Personalized Healthcare Solutions	85
		5.4.1 AI Chatbots for Patient Support and Education	85
		5.4.2 Real-Time and Telepatient Monitoring with Wearables	85
		5.4.3 Personalized Treatment Recommendations	86
		5.4.4 Predictive Models for Disease Progression and Risk Stratification	87
		5.4.5 Appointment Scheduling and Reminders	88
	5.5	Conclusion	90
	References		90
6	**AI to Empower People with Disabilities Communication and Autonomy**		97
	6.1	Introduction	97
	6.2	Communication Support	98
		6.2.1 Gesture Recognition	99
		6.2.2 Text Recognition	100
		6.2.3 Emotion Recognition	101
	6.3	Augmentative and Alternative Communication (AAC)	102
		6.3.1 Advanced AAC Systems	102
	6.4	AI Communication for Disabled Students	105
		6.4.1 Adaptive Learning	106
		6.4.2 Facial Expression	107
		6.4.3 Chat Robot	108
		6.4.4 Communication Assistant	108
		6.4.5 Interactive Robot	109
	6.5	Conclusion	109
	References		110

7 The Future of AI in Revolutionizing Support for Disabled Persons ... 115
- 7.1 Introduction ... 115
- 7.2 AI Redefining Independence for the Disabled ... 117
  - 7.2.1 Communication ... 117
  - 7.2.2 Educational Support ... 119
  - 7.2.3 Promoting an Independent Lifestyle ... 119
  - 7.2.4 Healthcare ... 120
  - 7.2.5 Smart Homes Promoting Independent Living ... 121
  - 7.2.6 Increasing Accessibility ... 122
  - 7.2.7 IOT for People with Disabilities ... 123
- 7.3 Visual Supports as Visual Language ... 124
  - 7.3.1 Augmented Reality Delivering Visual Supports ... 125
  - 7.3.2 Assistive AR/VR Developments ... 125
- 7.4 AI-Driven Autonomous Cars for Disability Mobility ... 126
  - 7.4.1 Pedestrian-Autonomous Vehicle Interaction ... 128
  - 7.4.2 Key Factors in Pedestrian-Autonomous Vehicle Communication ... 129
  - 7.4.3 Pedestrian Detection ... 129
- 7.5 Conclusion ... 130
- References ... 130

Chapter 1
Introduction to the Role of Artificial Intelligence in Disability Support

Abstract Artificial intelligence (AI) enables significant changes through which disabled individuals can achieve inclusion and obtain necessary resources more smoothly. AI-driven computer vision technology exhibits significant potential to aid those with impairments in vision, mobility, or voice. AI-powered solutions simplify everyday activities and improve personable capabilities through skill-enhancement and freedom-gaining features. AI technology in assistive tools improves societal acceptance which allows people with major physical challenges to maintain independent living. This chapter presents advanced AI solutions that transform daily life throughout different areas of human activity. AI technology used for cognitive support and object recognition as well as face recognition and speech recognition tools has enhanced overall usability for users. AI technology enables early disease identification combined with personalized medical interventions which improves healthcare delivery to patients. Restoring mobility to disabled people is now possible with the use of artificial intelligence (AI)-driven exoskeletons and devices. AI-based adaptive learning systems support educational accessibility because they enable students with disabilities to receive tailored personalized learning experiences at an open level. The improvements enabled by AI transformations redefine the concept of both independence and accessibility. The emerging world has the potential to fully integrate technology into daily life, which would give disabled people more freedom and opportunities to participate with others.

Keyword Artificial intelligence · Disabled · Assistance · Computer vision · Mobility independence

1.1 Introduction

Technology is increasingly influencing various aspects of modern life, reshaping the concept of mobility. Artificial intelligence (AI) is gradually transforming the challenges that people with disabilities faced in the past. This marks a thrilling beginning to a significant study exploring the collaboration between AI and disability to create a fairer future. Inclusivity progresses as society evolves. An increasing number of individuals with disabilities are exploring opportunities in the arts, education, employment, and social events. Two major challenges that have arisen during the process are constraints on space and restricted access to services and data. AI can significantly assist individuals with disabilities and transform their lives in remarkable ways (Collins et al., 2022; Dixon et al., 2022; Slee & Tait, 2022).

In the connection between AI and disability support, assistive tools are essential for breaking down barriers, empowering individuals with disabilities, and enhancing their overall quality of life. What sets AI-powered helpful technology apart is its emphasis on user-centered design. To cater to the needs and desires of individuals with disabilities, solutions are continually evolving and adapting according to user feedback. This method for continuous enhancement ensures that assistive devices align with users' aspirations and daily lives, all while fulfilling their practical requirements. Artificial intelligence (AI)-powered assistance is effective because it puts the needs of the user first and promotes involvement. This fosters autonomy and confidence in individuals with disabilities (Mao & Chang, 2023).

Artificial intelligence aims to train computers and other machines to think like people. Scientists are developing AI systems that leverage machine learning, data analytics, computer vision, and natural language processing to understand and learn from vast amounts of data. This indicates that AI can make smart choices and tackle challenges in ways that were once beyond the reach of everyday people. AI holds great promise in helping individuals find innovative solutions to the challenges faced by those with disabilities. The implementation and consideration of accessibility initiatives within the disability industry are significantly influenced by AI. Conventional approaches tend to concentrate on altering physical spaces or implementing minor adjustments, whereas AI-powered solutions provide tailored, personal assistance that transcends typical physical challenges. New developments in artificial intelligence have empowered people with disabilities, freeing them from the physical and mental barriers that once limited their ability to engage fully in society (Bricout et al., 2021; Givens & Morris, 2020; Morris, 2020).

A strong connection between AI and disability inclusion is on the horizon. There are many possible paths for future development, from creative assistive technologies that boost independence and well-being to healthcare improvements that enable personalized treatment and early diagnosis. As AI systems become more prevalent and sophisticated, individuals are meeting a wider array of AI-driven solutions designed to assist those with mental, physical, visual, or aural challenges in performing both ordinary and complicated tasks. Researchers assert that enhancing the accessibility of AI technology can profoundly impact the lives of individuals with disabilities across several industries. This chapter offers a comprehensive examination of the fundamental qualities underpinning AI-driven solutions for disabilities.

1.2 Disabled Person Assistance with AI

The importance of people feeling connected to one another is growing in today's fast-paced, globally connected world. Fortunately, new ways for people with impairments to interact with their surroundings have emerged because of AI technology (Huq et al., 2024; Karn et al., 2024). Multiple aspects are involved in the adaptation of technologies for those with disabilities. They may possess diverse resources, including dexterity, mobility, confidence, processing speed, attention, health, memory, technical competence, motivation, knowledge, experience, and visual, aural, and kinesthetic abilities. Proficiency in reading comprehension, written expression, efficient communication, time and financial management, and fundamental mathematical and statistical skills, among other life competencies, may be necessary. A diverse array of resources is accessible to them, including training, peer support, professional counsel, technical assistance, and financial support. They are present in various environments and utilize an extensive array of tools, including but not limited to: text-to-speech and e-reading software, word processors and proofreading applications, visual mapping and planning instruments, reminders, speech recognition technologies, mathematical and computational aids, study resources, environmental controls and alarms, wearable technology, and communication devices (Radanliev et al., 2024). A mobile phone is one example of a technology that might offer numerous customization choices to accommodate individuals with disabilities. This technology enables users to select the settings that best suit their needs. This chapter analyzes various AI-assisted systems, encompassing those that support mobility, cognition, computer vision, and speech recognition. A significant shift is underway in disability support because of the emergence of AI-driven assistive devices. These enhancements are uplifting the lives of individuals with disabilities by eliminating obstacles, fostering independence, and boosting their overall well-being (Morina et al., 2024).

1.3 AI-Based Computer Vision for Assistive Technology Tasks

People with disabilities can take advantage of various AI-powered tools that utilize computer vision methods (Fig. 1.1) (Sahoo & Choudhury, 2024).

1.3.1 Object Recognition

In computer vision, AI algorithms can help discover and categorize objects in the real world. This is especially advantageous for blind persons or having impaired vision, as it facilitates navigation and improves their engagement with the world. Object recognition systems enhance the understanding of the environment by providing

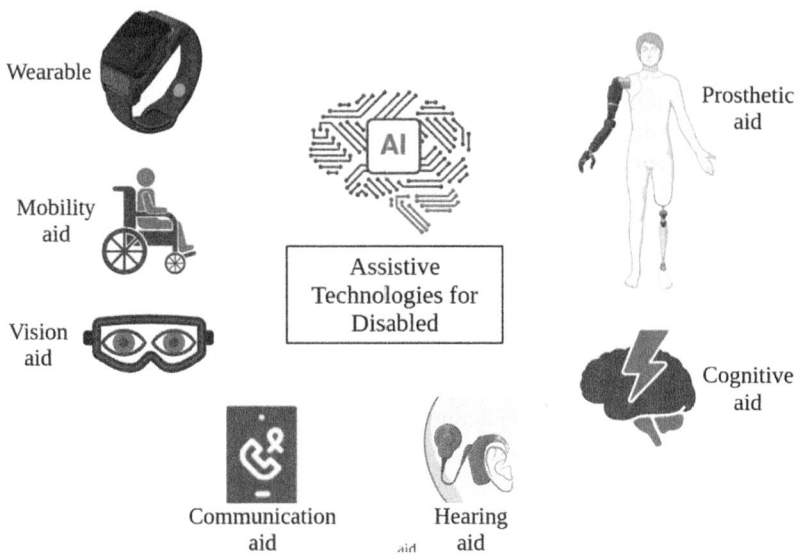

Fig. 1.1 Various AI-powered tools utilize AI-based assistive technologies for the disabled

audio descriptions of nearby objects. Object recognition is a fascinating application of assistive technology that utilizes artificial intelligence to support individuals with disabilities (Aung et al., 2024). The primary objective is to increase environmental awareness. AI can spot objects, allowing systems to play audio descriptions of what's nearby, helping users grasp their environment more effectively. This may be especially beneficial for persons experiencing visual impairments or other difficulties that hinder mobility (Dang et al., 2024). Object recognition algorithms help people understand the things they see by identifying and categorizing them. When an object recognition system detects a table or chair, it may provide audio details about the shape, size, and position of the item (Souza et al., 2024).

The provision of assistance in navigation is available once it has been established. Combining object recognition systems with assistive technologies, particularly AI-driven navigation tools, enhances the accuracy and reliability of the information provided to users about their environment. An object recognition system can help a blind person or someone with low vision get around in a busy area by finding obstacles and help them to get around (Abidi et al., 2024). Additionally, it pertains to the proper management of objects. Artificial intelligence (AI)-based object identification systems might alleviate mobility issues for certain individuals. An identification system assists individuals in monitoring their belongings by identifying typical household goods and providing auditory signals regarding their location and orientation.

1.3.2 Facial Recognition

Face recognition systems that use AI can identify people and give them personalized help. After authenticating a user, an AI-powered face recognition system might give them personalized spoken directions about finding their way around in a public place like a museum or shopping mall. In many ways, facial recognition can make assistance technology better (Alamirew & Kebede, 2024). At first, AI-powered face recognition systems can improve access control by letting only authorized people safely enter certain areas, devices, or resources. It is easier for people with disabilities to use AI-based face recognition technology instead of traditional ways of identifying themselves, like passwords or keycards. Subsequently, AI-driven mood detection systems will employ facial recognition technology to ascertain individuals' emotional states. This will let assistive devices give better help. An emotion recognition system could instantly pick up on worries and tensions and then suggest ways to relax or deal with them (Chhimpa et al., 2024). Face recognition technology built on AI can also be used to make the user experience better for people with disabilities. Assistive technology that uses facial recognition can know each user and give them personalized help based on their choices and needs (Ghafoor et al., 2024).

AI-based facial recognition systems can help people with autism and other communication issues by reading their feelings from their faces. This can assist individuals with speech difficulties in comprehending others and vice versa (Adako et al., 2024). Blind individuals or those having visual impairments can utilize AI-driven navigation systems and facial recognition technologies to assist them in navigating unfamiliar environments. Facial recognition technology can assist visually impaired individuals in navigating busy environments by promptly locating and recognizing individuals, providing auditory cues regarding their positions and directions to reach them (Feghali et al., 2024). Face recognition technology that is built on AI can help people with disabilities a lot. Face recognition technologies can give accurate and reliable information about nearby people, which can help disabled people live on their own with more confidence and independence.

1.3.3 Gaze Detection

AI-driven automated algorithms capable of detecting gaze can monitor the user's eye movements and provide feedback on their focus of attention. People having trouble moving around can benefit from this technology because it lets them handle their assistive equipment only by moving their eyes (Hsieh et al., 2024). There are several ways that gaze recognition can improve assistive technology. AI-based gaze detection technologies can help people with neurological diseases like cerebral palsy or amyotrophic lateral sclerosis (ALS) communicate a lot better. Gaze detection systems are a type of assistive technology that let blind people or have low vision use a computer or other devices to choose letters or words. This improves augmentative and alternative communication (AAC) (Megalingam et al., 2024).

Individuals with mobility challenges, such as quadriplegics, can receive assistance navigating their surroundings through AI-driven gaze recognition technology. Gaze detection systems enhance the independence of wheelchairs and other assistive devices by interpreting where the user is looking (Manzoor et al., 2024). As a result, automated gaze detection technology can help assess the level of attention in individuals with cognitive challenges, such as autism or attention deficit hyperactivity disorder (ADHD). Gaze detection systems can track eye movement to determine if a user is focused on a specific item (Sakthimohan et al., 2024). The use of AI-based gaze detection systems improves environmental management by enabling those with impairments to operate devices such as temperature and lighting controls. Gaze detection systems are designed to facilitate interaction with the environment by using the user's gaze direction as input (Kahlon et al., 2024). People with disabilities can benefit greatly from gaze recognition in many ways. Gaze detection systems offer a new way to interact with the world and get more people involved in different activities.

1.4 Additional AI Assistive Technology

1.4.1 Speech Recognition

Voice recognition is an important part of AI-driven assistive tools. Speech recognition systems provide a novel alternative for those with movement disabilities or disorders that hinder conventional communication methods, enabling contact with technology. These technologies allow individuals to control objects, engage in real-time conversations, navigate computer interfaces, and produce text by transcribing spoken words into written form or commands (Abhishek et al., 2022; Debnath et al., 2023; Irugalbandara et al., 2022; Yang et al., 2023). This unique communication medium enhances a deeper sense of belonging in professional and social contexts, while also augmenting their ability to express their thoughts and ideas. Speech recognition also assists those with writing difficulties in utilizing their speech for composition. It can also aid individuals with hearing impairments by offering subtitles and transcripts. Initially, speech recognition was customized to the specific needs of each user through extensive local training.

However, AI-based speech recognition has become increasingly popular because of advanced software-based speech recognition (Baibhav, 2024). Development of speech recognition, speech synthesis, or machine translation for disabled can be made possible due to AI-based algorithms. Additionally, a specialized system is required for individuals with dysarthric speech, as conventional speech recognition is ineffective (Alhinti et al., 2023). The application of AI in lipreading has demonstrated an

1.4 Additional AI Assistive Technology

enhancement in the precision of speech recognition, particularly in noisy environments (Assael et al., 2016). The increasing accessibility and decreasing cost of 3D cameras should further enhance accuracy (de Silva et al., 2014). Numerous individuals have articulated apprehensions over "Deepfakes," wherein artificial intelligence has been employed to manipulate individuals' lip movements and speech, rendering them to seemingly utter statements they never made (Yan, 2022). Nevertheless, it seems that no one has considered employing the same technology to enhance individuals' lipreading capabilities. Automatic captions can denote some non-verbal noises (e.g., music, laughter, and clapping (Hoffman & Friedman, 2018), while advancements in emotion detection from speech and facial expressions are progressing. A customized voice can be created for persons at danger of voice loss due to impending illness (Westley et al., 2019). Overall speech recognition by AI for disabled is a great tool that could enhance the involvement of disabled person with the surrounding.

1.4.2 Facilitating Communication

Artificial intelligence (AI) has emerged as a transformative tool in facilitating communication for individuals with disabilities, enabling greater inclusion and accessibility in everyday life. Through innovative applications, AI-powered solutions are breaking communication barriers for people with speech, hearing, and motor impairments. For instance, speech-to-text and text-to-speech technologies empower individuals with hearing or speech disabilities to engage seamlessly in conversations (Regondi et al., 2025). Similarly, advanced natural language processing (NLP) algorithms drive real-time sign language translation, converting gestures into spoken or written language, and vice versa. Artificial intelligence supports individuals with mobility challenges by offering adaptive interfaces that enhance communication through eye-tracking, brain-computer interfaces (BCI), and predictive text technologies (Deodhare, 2015). These technologies enhance autonomy, enabling users to communicate their thoughts effectively even with restricted physical mobility.

Assistive technology powered by artificial intelligence, such as voice-activated smart assistants, facilitates daily interactions and aids individuals with disabilities in communicating with their environment. People with disabilities find it easier to interact with artificial intelligence speech technologies, such as Alexa, Siri, and Echo. Visually impaired people can use these apps to turn text and pictures into spoken words. Cognitively impaired people can use text-to-speech technology to improve their communication and comprehension of written material (Orynbay et al., 2024). People having trouble speaking can now use Google's Parrotron, an AI app that can turn their slurred words into dialogue that is easy to understand. These AI technologies can help experts make technology that is more open and collaborative for people with a wide range of disabilities.

Also, personalized AI models made from user profiles adapt to different situations, making sure that the interpretation and reaction are correct. Putting artificial intelligence into assistive and alternative communication devices has opened up new options for people having trouble in communicating, giving them faster and more natural ways to express themselves. These technologies can help people with disabilities feel more included in group situations and improve communication with others by letting them transcribe speech in high quality (Chemnad & Othman, 2024). Businesses can also provide better customer service by using voice technology that is driven by AI. Chatbots that use artificial intelligence (AI) can help customer service reps talk to disabled customers, better understanding their needs and better meeting those needs (Khamaj, 2025). Additionally, this promotes the creation of better experiences, which could lead to more loyal customers, especially those with disabilities. AI promotes social inclusion by facilitating participation in education, employment, and social activities, thereby reducing stigma and improving the quality of life for millions, in addition to technical advancements. As AI continues to evolve, its potential to revolutionize communication for disabled individuals underscores its pivotal role in creating a more inclusive and equitable society.

1.4.3 Vision Technology for Mobility Independence

The ability to move about freely is fundamental to independence, and assistive technology that uses artificial intelligence is revolutionizing life for people with mobility challenges. These technologies offer individualized resolutions to mobility problems by combining data from sensors with machine learning algorithms. Innovations such as adaptive smart wheelchairs that negotiate intricate surroundings (Kumar & Jain, 2022; Pydala et al., 2023; Walle et al., 2022) and exoskeletons that improve mobility (Lin et al., 2023; Satyavathi et al., 2023) promote autonomy and enable persons to participate in a broader spectrum of activities with assurance. Artificial intelligence (AI) can facilitate autonomous mobility, as illustrated in Fig. 1.1. Additionally, advancements in computer vision technology constitute a transformational aspect of AI-driven help. This enables visually challenged folks to interact with and traverse their environment. Applications powered by AI combine image identification, object detection, and scene analysis to help with autonomous navigation, obstacle detection, and real-time environmental descriptions (Bharath, 2022; Patthanajitsilp & Chongstitvatana, 2022; Valipoor & Antonio, 2023; Yang et al., 2022). This modern visual comprehension enables individuals to autonomously navigate environments, recognize things, and interact with their surroundings in previously unattainable manners. Possible uses of AI for people with visual impairments are depicted in Fig. 1.1.

1.4.4 Autonomous Vehicles

Artificial intelligence-controlled robotic vehicles are transforming mobility for individuals with disabilities, enhancing their independence, safety, and accessibility to

1.4 Additional AI Assistive Technology

necessary destinations. Computer vision, machine learning, and real-time sensor data are some of the advanced technologies that these cars use to find their way and drive themselves. Autonomous vehicles take away the need for people with physical limitations to drive by hand, letting them move on their own using voice commands or mobile apps. This technology uses advanced algorithms to spot obstacles, recognize traffic lights, and discover the best routes, ensuring travel is both safe and speedy. Automated wheelchair ramps, adjustable seats, and simple controls enhance accessibility, making these cars a great option for those with mobility challenges. LiDAR, radar, and GPS technologies assist blind individuals or having low vision in navigating with greater precision, while audio feedback enhances their awareness of the environment around them. Similarly, AI systems that provide individualized learning, real-time assistance, and reminders to address the particular requirements of individuals with cognitive impairments are beneficial to such individuals. Autonomous cars powered by AI not only help individuals, but they also make society better by allowing disabled people to use public and shared transportation systems. These cars are very important for getting people where they need to go, especially in places like poor or rural areas where public transportation may not be very convenient. AI-driven mobility solutions enhance the autonomy of individuals with disabilities by decreasing reliance on caregivers or specialized services, thereby facilitating greater access to education, employment, healthcare, and social activities. As advancements in autonomous vehicle technology continue, they hold immense potential to redefine transportation accessibility and foster greater inclusion in society (Phutthammawong et al., 2020; Treviranus, 2017).

1.4.5 Autonomy-Promoting Cognitive Support

AI-enabled cognitive support is transforming the way individuals with cognitive disabilities achieve greater autonomy, fostering their ability to manage tasks, make decisions, and lead independent lives. Through advanced technologies such as machine learning, natural language processing, and personalized algorithms, AI systems are tailored to address the unique needs of individuals with challenges in memory, attention, learning, or decision-making. Cognitive assistive tools powered by AI provide real-time guidance and reminders, helping users manage schedules, medications, and daily activities effectively. These tools adapt to individual learning patterns and preferences, ensuring a personalized experience that evolves with the user's needs. Difficulty with everyday tasks and speech are hallmarks of cognitive impairments. To improve communication, memory recall, and decision-making, cognitive support systems powered by AI use machine learning and natural language processing. These technological advancements have the potential to improve time management, send out reminders, and provide discussion replies that are relevant to the current environment (Afonso-Jaco & Katz, 2022; Boulanger, 2022; Wieseler, 2022). These technologies increase personal liberty and allow people to actively participate in their everyday routines and social life by bridging the knowledge gap.

Additionally, AI-powered speech recognition and contextual reasoning aid in simplifying complex information, enabling individuals to process and comprehend tasks at their own pace. Virtual assistants and chatbots provide 24/7 support, offering step-by-step instructions, decision-making aids, or emotional reassurance during challenging situations. AI-driven social cognition solutions help individuals with conditions such as autism or traumatic brain injuries to understand social cues, thereby enhancing their communication and interaction skills. Additionally, wearable devices integrated with AI sensors assess cognitive states in real time, providing insights and preventative interventions during episodes of disorientation or stress. These technologies enable individuals to traverse settings, seek knowledge, and engage in professional and social endeavors with assurance. By diminishing dependence on caretakers and fostering self-sufficiency, AI-driven cognitive support cultivates cognitive autonomy and improves overall quality of life, facilitating a more inclusive society in which individuals with cognitive disabilities can flourish independently.

1.4.6 Localization

AI-driven localization is transforming accessibility for those with disabilities, enabling them to explore and engage with their environment more autonomously. Utilizing technologies such as computer vision, GPS, and machine learning, AI-driven solutions deliver real-time location data and context-sensitive support. For visually impaired individuals, AI-powered navigation apps and wearable devices use audio cues or haptic feedback to guide them safely through unfamiliar environments, identifying obstacles, landmarks, and safe routes. Similarly, individuals with hearing impairments benefit from real-time text or visual alerts that enhance spatial awareness and communication. Localization is also defined as "the process of modifying a product or service to be more suitable for a particular country, region, locale, or individual" (Wen et al., 2024). Is localization synonymous with "personalization" for a cultural group? Assistive devices may require localization in both linguistic and cultural contexts. Due to the inappropriacy of many symbols and the absence of certain cultural symbols, researchers developed specialized symbols to aid individuals with verbal or written communication difficulties (Nedjar & M'hamedi, 2024). A graphic designer would work closely with symbol users to create these symbols, which would be a laborious and expensive production procedure. However, researchers are presently exploring new methods for the automatic generation of symbols from photos using AI.

Selecting the appropriate symbol from a symbol board that is organized hierarchically can be a time-consuming process. For instance, choosing foods from the primary category, vegetables from the secondary category, and cauliflower from the vegetable subcategory. Automatically discerning the necessary symbols according to the context would enhance efficiency (Khan, 2024). For instance, if the system recognizes that the user is in a retail environment and is aware of their shopping list, it would operate efficiently. Also, artificial intelligence-powered indoor localization technologies like beacon technology and virtual reality make it easier for people to find their way around places like hospitals, shopping malls, and airports. These technologies also help people with cognitive problems find their way around by making travel easier and more efficient. Localization powered by AI gets rid of physical and spatial barriers, giving disabled people more freedom, inclusion, and movement, which improves their quality of life and social integration.

1.5 New Developments in Healthcare

There have been big improvements in early diagnosis, personalized treatment plans, and rehabilitation for disabled people since artificial intelligence (AI) was introduced to healthcare (Khalid et al., 2024). There are a lot of new possibilities coming up now that AI is being used in healthcare, especially when it comes to helping people with disabilities. Artificial intelligence is transforming healthcare by enabling personalized care for patients, facilitating earlier diagnoses, and providing specialized treatments for individuals with disabilities. This section examines the capacity of artificial intelligence to revolutionize healthcare, specifically in augmenting the welfare of individuals with disabilities through enhanced diagnostic precision, the formulation of more efficacious treatment strategies, and the overall improvement of health outcomes (Fig. 1.2).

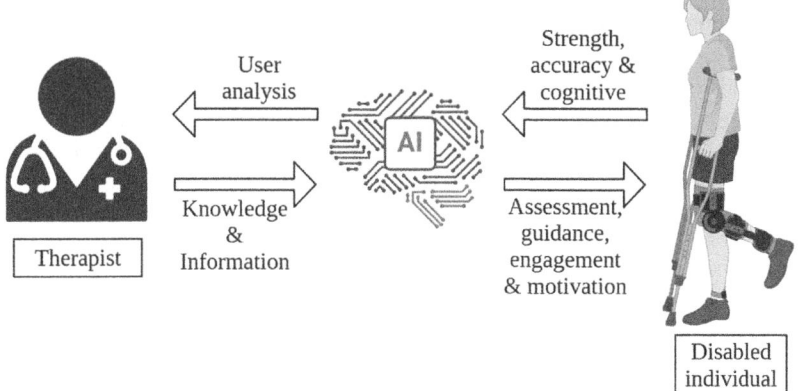

Fig. 1.2 Role of AI to transform healthcare of individuals with disabilities by improving diagnostic accuracy, developing more effective treatment plans, and overall elevating health outcomes

1.5.1 Precision Diagnosis

AI-driven precision diagnosis is transforming healthcare for individuals with disabilities by delivering tailored, accurate, and swift medical insights that significantly enhance care and quality of life. AI systems excel at spotting health issues by utilizing advanced machine learning techniques and data analysis, while also integrating various types of medical information such as imaging, genetic profiles, and clinical records. This is particularly beneficial for individuals with disabilities, as their distinct health issues or atypical symptoms can complicate standard diagnostic approaches. In the realm of assisting individuals with disabilities, AI plays a crucial role in providing precise diagnoses. Artificial intelligence systems can explore large and complex medical datasets to uncover trends and issues that might be overlooked by other approaches (Arumugam et al., 2022; Khoury et al., 2022; Wickramasinghe et al., 2022). Artificial intelligence (AI) enhances the accuracy of diagnoses by examining intricate links in medical data, reducing the likelihood of errors, and accelerating the delivery of effective treatments for patients (Furini et al., 2022; Kem, 2022; Yu et al., 2022).

AI-driven tools, such as medical imaging systems, can detect early signs of diseases like neural issues, musculoskeletal limitations, or heart conditions, allowing for prompt treatment. Moreover, wearable technology powered by AI continuously monitors key health indicators and provides instant alerts for emergencies such as seizures, falls, or irregular heart rhythms, often seen in individuals with impairments. AI-driven prediction models analyze health data to identify trends and anticipate future issues. This allows doctors to create tailored treatment plans and minimize risks efficiently. These tools assist doctors in improving diagnoses and reducing hospital visits, promoting a more proactive approach to healthcare. AI addresses various health issues simultaneously and provides comprehensive information, ensuring that individuals with disabilities receive personalized, in-depth care tailored to their unique needs. AI in healthcare helps individuals manage their health more easily, fostering independence and self-reliance. As AI improves, its ability to make precise diagnoses will play a crucial role in transforming disability healthcare, reducing disparities, and opening doors to a future of tailored and accessible medical care.

1.5.2 Personalized Treatment Plans

One area where AI is making an impact, beyond basic diagnosis, is in personalized therapy options. AI-driven personalized treatment plans are transforming medical care for individuals with disabilities by offering precise, tailored, and adaptable solutions that cater to their unique needs. Artificial intelligence systems can enhance therapy by analyzing a person's health data, genetic markers, and treatment responses. Individuals with impairments require additional support due to their distinct medical needs, often leading to the necessity for personalized treatment plans.

AI systems use machine learning and data analytics to examine a person's medical history, genetic details, lifestyle habits, and real-time health metrics to create tailored treatment options. This approach considers both health conditions and particular functional challenges, which are among the various and often complex healthcare issues encountered by individuals with disabilities. AI-powered solutions continuously monitor health changes and change therapies in real time to enhance outcomes and minimize adverse effects. AI assists doctors in developing tailored treatment plans for every patient, focusing on medication management and physical therapy that align with their unique needs and objectives (Barua et al., 2022; Piette et al., 2022; Sahal et al., 2022). Moreover, wearable devices powered by AI provide instant feedback, helping to facilitate adjustments in medication dosages or rehabilitation exercises. These approaches help healthcare professionals collaborate more effectively, resulting in improved patient care. Personalized treatment plans powered by AI provide precision, speed, and flexibility, empowering individuals with disabilities to take charge of their health and enhancing their independence and overall quality of life.

1.5.3 Rehabilitation and Prosthetics

The advancement of prosthetics and rehabilitation is being facilitated by artificial intelligence, creating new opportunities for individuals experiencing difficulty with their musculature or mobility (Fig. 1.3). Rehabilitation and AI-driven prosthetics are transforming the way individuals with disabilities regain their mobility, independence, and overall quality of life. In rehabilitation, AI systems harness smart machine learning and real-time data to craft tailored therapy plans. These programs are designed to meet the unique needs of each individual with a disability, adapting as they grow to ensure optimal outcomes. Exoskeletons and robotic rehab systems powered by AI assist patients in recovering their motor skills by guiding their movements accurately and providing feedback throughout therapy sessions.

AI-driven exoskeletons and prosthetic limbs can replicate an individual's natural gait and offer natural support. Also, AI-enhanced rehabilitation systems make it easier to change treatment plans based on progress, which leads to a faster and more effective healing (Malcangi, 2021; Nayak & Das, 2020; Shahabi et al., 2022). When virtual reality (VR) and artificial intelligence (AI) are combined, they create immersive environments for cognitive and physical rehabilitation. This makes treatment both relaxing and very effective. AI speeds up recovery, lowers the length of therapy, and makes sure that each person reaches their full potential by tracking their performance and making changes in real time. Artificial intelligence is driving progress in prosthetics by making artificial systems that are more complex, adaptable, and smart. Modern prosthetics that are powered by AI use sensors, neural interfaces, and machine learning to move like a real leg and change based on what the user wants. These prosthetics improve usefulness, letting amputees walk, run, or do difficult tasks

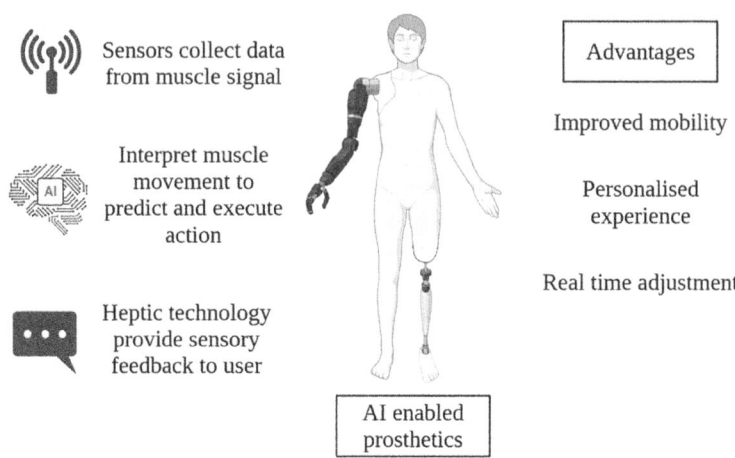

Fig. 1.3 AI-enabled prosthetics and rehabilitation, creating new opportunities for disabled individuals experiencing difficulty with their musculature or mobility

accurately. When AI is added to myoelectric prosthetics, it can read muscle signals and turn them into complex movements, which makes control smooth.

This personalized method not only speeds up recovery, but it also makes it easier for people to do things on their own (Fig. 1.3). Furthermore, AI algorithms continuously learn from user interactions, enhancing their efficiency and user-friendliness over time. These changes make it possible for disabled people to regain their independence and feel safe doing normal things. As AI technology improves, it has the potential to greatly change rehabilitation and prosthetics, making the future more open and available to everyone.

1.6 Inclusive Education

Inclusive education ensures that all students, regardless of their background, intellectual capacity, or disabilities, have equal opportunities to get a quality education. AI makes inclusive education much better by providing a wide range of tools and solutions that can be tailored to each student's specific learning needs. It helps people talk to each other better and gets more people involved, especially kids with disabilities (Rehan, 2023). AI-driven inclusive education is changing the way people with disabilities learn by making learning more available, personalized, and interesting. Speech-to-text apps, text-to-speech systems, and real-time sign language speakers are all examples of AI-powered solutions that help students having trouble speaking, hearing, or seeing communicate better. Adaptive learning platforms look at each student's learning style and needs and make lesson plans and pacing that work with their cognitive and physical limitations. Artificial intelligence-powered

1.6 Inclusive Education

assistive technology, like virtual tutors and smart classroom gadgets, keeps students interested and helps them learn all the time. AI improves accessibility, interest, and fairness, which helps students with disabilities do well in schools that are open to everyone. This section will examine the impact of artificial intelligence on education, emphasizing its role in facilitating communication and connection for students with disabilities, as well as enhancing the flexibility of learning pathways.

1.6.1 Learning Opportunities

Individuals, independent of their abilities, have the right to equal access to all services. The use of artificial intelligence (AI) could help make inclusion better. Braille enables visually impaired individuals to read, much like subtitles aid individuals with hearing impairments in understanding a video. Artificial intelligence-driven educational choices are making things better for people with disabilities by making learning more accessible, personalized, and open to everyone. Adaptive learning tools, virtual tutors, and assistive technology are all examples of AI-powered products that help students with a wide range of learning needs by providing personalized lesson plans and quick help. For example, blind people or having low vision can now use online Braille teaching programs that are run by AI, which gives them more educational options (Ali, 2023). Optical character recognition (OCR) is used in these programs to turn tactile Braille text into digital files.

Speech-to-text, text-to-speech, and AI-driven sign language tools help kids having trouble hearing, seeing, or speaking communicate better. Through the use of interactive learning tools and virtual environments, artificial intelligence makes participation higher. This makes education more effective and open to everyone. By addressing particular challenges and fostering equity, AI ensures that students with disabilities can achieve quality education and reach their full potential. Additionally, professionals around the globe can develop a growth mindset by adopting AI-driven solutions. Customized learning paths can be developed to assist individuals with disabilities in recognizing appropriate training programs and resources that align with their skills. Individuals can also gain from ongoing performance feedback through AI methodologies, enabling them to learn from their errors (Trewin et al., 2019).

Furthermore, artificial intelligence (AI) solutions assist researchers in identifying skill deficiencies in an individual assisting in competencies, and developing targeted training programs to facilitate professional development for disabled individual (Kumar et al., 2023). Utilizing AR and VR to develop immersive educational settings for disabled is a feasible alternative. Also, organizations must guarantee that employees with disabilities get tailored training programs that equip them with the requisite knowledge and skills to perform their duties effectively (Mastam & Zaharudin, 2024). This fosters a varied workforce that empowers each individual. Companies can enhance their profitability by cultivating a growth mindset among their employees through unbiased and successful execution.

1.6.2 Pathways to Personalized Education

AI-enabled personalized learning pathways and language processing tools are revolutionizing education, creating tailored learning experiences, and overcoming communication barriers for disabled individuals. Artificial intelligence (AI) systems evaluate the strengths, weaknesses, and preferences of pupils or individuals with impairments to create personalized learning pathways through the use of sophisticated machine learning algorithms. These adaptive platforms change the pace, difficulty, and material in real time, making sure that each student gets guidance that is just right for them. Customized pathways that offer resources in easy-to-use forms, such as audio, visual aids, or simplified text, can help people having cognitive or physical limitations become more engaged and understand what they are reading.

Language processing tools powered by AI can assist students facing different communication challenges. This area includes technologies like voice recognition software, language translation apps, and text-to-speech systems. Speech recognition tools make it easier for students having trouble hearing or speaking to talk to each other. Also, language processing methods that are powered by AI, like natural language processing (NLP), make things a lot easier for everyone to use. Speech-to-text technologies help people having trouble hearing or speaking turn spoken language into written text. Text-to-speech technologies help blind people or having low vision in learning by turning written material into audio versions.

Text-to-speech technology also makes written material available to students having trouble seeing or reading (Ingavélez-Guerra et al., 2022; Sharma & Dash, 2023; Zdravkova, 2022). Real-time translation services provided by artificial intelligence (AI) make it easier for students speaking different languages or use sign language to talk to each other. Artificial intelligence could be used in the classroom to help kids with disabilities. AI-driven systems can rapidly translate languages, facilitating participation for non-native speakers or people that struggle with language acquisition. These technologies make it easier to understand complicated language, which helps people with cognitive problems understand and interact with educational material better. AI gets rid of barriers in standard education systems by combining personalized learning paths and language processing technologies. This makes sure that all students have the same chances to learn. This method makes sure that education is open to everyone, easy to get to, and fits different needs. It also lets students learn at their own pace and in the way that works best for them. As AI gets better, it will be used in schools to make the learning setting more fair, flexible, and helpful for everyone (Fosch-Villaronga & Poulsen, 2022; Siregar et al., 2023; Skowronek et al., 2022).

1.6.3 Revolutionizing Communication and Interaction

Communication and engagement in education are changing because of AI, which is making learning more open, accessible, and interesting for students all over the world. Artificial intelligence (AI)-powered technologies like natural language processing (NLP), speech recognition, and real-time translation are making it easier for learners with a wide range of needs, especially those with challenges, to communicate. Speech-to-text and text-to-speech technology facilitates seamless access to and interaction with educational information for students with hearing, speech, or visual impairments. Children with impairments now engage with their peers and educators in significantly altered ways due to AI-enhanced communication technology. Students with disabilities facing challenges in speech or mobility can employ software and devices augmented by artificial intelligence to boost communication using symbols, text, or eye-tracking technology. Real-time language translation systems facilitate comprehension for multilingual learners, enabling them full participation in classroom activities.

Furthermore, children with hearing loss or deafness can improve their communication with AI-powered sign language identification and interpretation systems (Hughes et al., 2022; Zdravkova et al., 2022). These technologies eliminate barriers to communication, enabling students with disabilities to engage effectively in classroom discussions and collaborative activities. AI-powered chatbots and virtual assistants enhance communication by providing responses to inquiries, offering personalized guidance, and delivering round-the-clock support. Adaptive learning systems utilize artificial intelligence to analyze individual students' learning styles and requirements, thus personalizing the delivery of content and the manner in which students are engaged. This makes it easier for teachers and students to talk to each other. AI-powered collaboration tools also make it easy for students to connect with each other in real and virtual classrooms, which improves teamwork and student engagement.

Incorporating artificial intelligence into inclusive education has the potential to revolutionize it in numerous ways. It helps kids with disabilities communicate and be more involved, gives teachers the tools they need to make personalized programs, and gives people with disabilities language processing tools to help them. When AI technologies are used in education, they make it more interesting, dynamic, and fair by making it easier for students of all types to communicate, learn, and grow. Not only does this change make learning better, it also makes the school a better place for everyone, giving every student the tools and help they need to do well in school. Leveraging AI's capabilities, inclusive education can achieve its objective of providing disabled students, irrespective of their type of disability, with equitable access to a high-quality education.

1.7 AI Promoting Disabled Independence

AI is transforming the lives of individuals with disabilities by promoting independence and enabling them to lead empowered lifestyles. More and more, opportunities for people with impairments to live independently in their personal and professional life are opening up because of artificial intelligence (Abedi et al., 2024). Through innovative applications and adaptive technologies, AI addresses various challenges, from mobility and communication to daily living and healthcare management. AI-powered personal assistants, such as smart speakers and mobile apps, simplify routine tasks by enabling voice-activated control over household appliances, reminders, and schedules.

Virtual assistants like Google Assistant and Amazon Alexa can automate a variety of voice actions and send reminders; many AI applications help disabled perform efficient workflows with these tools. Disabled have the opportunity to enhance their workforce with AI-powered chatbots that can assist with a wide range of tasks. These tools allow individuals with physical or cognitive disabilities to manage their homes and lives independently. Automation of repetitive tasks through robotic process automation (RPA), personalized data suggestions generated by AI-integrated recommendation systems, and visual data identification and interpretation through object detection, image recognition, face recognition, and quality control are all additional AI tools that can improve workflow for disabled (Ghulaxe, 2024).

In the realm of mobility, AI-enabled navigation apps provide real-time guidance, helping visually impaired users safely navigate their surroundings. Autonomous vehicles powered by AI provide exceptional freedom for individuals with physical disabilities, allowing them to move independently without needing caregivers or conventional transportation. Wearable devices powered by AI monitor health metrics and provide quick alerts for emergencies, encouraging independence in managing health. Additionally, innovative communication tools like AI-powered speech-to-text apps and live sign language interpreters improve interaction for those with hearing or speech challenges. Additionally, all employees facing challenges in the workplace can use these technologies to boost their productivity, cutting down on tedious manual tasks and allowing more attention to important duties. This can help executives with challenges to clear away obstacles in their workflow, making it easier to carry out and finish their tasks (Rojas et al., 2024). AI improves functionality by customizing solutions to specific needs, boosting confidence and inclusion, and enabling individuals with disabilities to engage fully in education, work, and social activities. The development of AI demonstrates its capacity to foster autonomy and its revolutionary potential to build a more equal and welcoming society.

1.8 Conclusion

Artificial intelligence has emerged as a promising technology for assistive devices that can aid those with disabilities in their daily activities. AI-enabled computer vision techniques can enhance autonomy and independence for those with disabilities. AI-enabled assistive technologies, including object identification, facial recognition, speech recognition, cognitive assistance, and AI-driven healthcare utilizing early disease detection algorithms, have led to substantial advancements. Moreover, AI-enhanced prosthetics and exoskeletons could significantly enhance mobility for individuals with limb disabilities. AI has the potential to transform education by developing inclusive learning environments that accommodate different learning styles, hence facilitating academic success for children with impairments.

References

Abedi, A., Colella, T. J., Pakosh, M., & Khan, S. S. (2024). Artificial intelligence-driven virtual rehabilitation for people living in the community: A scoping review. *NPJ Digital Medicine, 7*(1), 25.

Abhishek, S., Sathish, H., Kumar, A., & Anjali, T. (2022). Aiding the visually impaired using artificial intelligence and speech recognition technology. In *2022 4th International Conference on Inventive Research in Computing Applications (ICIRCA)* (pp. 1356–1362). IEEE.

Abidi, M. H., Siddiquee, A. N., Alkhalefah, H., & Srivastava, V. (2024). *A comprehensive review of navigation systems for visually impaired individuals.* Heliyon. Volume 10, Issue 11, 19.

Adako, O., Adeusi, O., & Alaba, P. (2024). Integrating AI tools for enhanced autism education: A comprehensive review. *International Journal of Developmental Disabilities*, 1–3.

Afonso-Jaco, A., & Katz, B. F. (2022). Spatial knowledge via auditory information for blind individuals: Spatial cognition studies and the use of audio-VR. *Sensors, 22*(13), 4794.

Alamirew, S. G., & Kebede, G. A. (2024). *Developing an assistive technology for visually impaired persons: Ethiopian currency identification.* Available at SSRN 4697484.

Alhinti, L., Cunningham, S., & Christensen, H. (2023). The Dysarthric expressed emotional database (DEED): An audio-visual database in British English. *PLoS ONE, 18*(8), e0287971.

Ali, S. A. (2023). Artificial intelligence techniques to understand braille: a language for visually impaired individuals. In *Handbook of research on artificial intelligence applications in literary works and social media* (pp. 254–276). IGI Global.

Arumugam, D., Govindaraju, K., & Tamilarasan, A. K. (2022, February 3). AIIoT-based smart framework for screening specific learning disabilities. In *Machine learning for critical internet of medical things: Applications and use cases* (pp. 103–124). Springer International Publishing.

Assael, Y. M., Shillingford, B., Whiteson, S., & De Freitas, N. (2016, November 5). *Lipnet: End-to-end sentence-level lipreading.* arXiv:1611.01599

Aung, M. M., Maneetham, D., Crisnapati, P. N., & Thwe, Y. (2024). *Enhancing object recognition for visually impaired individuals using computer vision.*

Baibhav, A. (2024, August 25). Artificial intelligence & its relevance in blended learning. In *Artificial intelligence in education* (p. 312).

Barua, P. D., Vicnesh, J., Gururajan, R., Oh, S. L., Palmer, E., Azizan, M. M., Kadri, N. A., & Acharya, U. R. (2022). Artificial intelligence enabled personalised assistive tools to enhance education of children with neurodevelopmental disorders—A review. *International Journal of Environmental Research and Public Health, 19*(3), 1192.

Bharath, M. R. (2022). Controlling mouse and virtual keyboard using eye-tracking by computer vision. *Journal of Algebraic Statistics, 13*(3), 3354–3368.

Boulanger, J. (2022). *Ways of knowing, ways of being: Exploring a good life through participatory audio/visual methods with people labelled with an intellectual disability* (Doctoral dissertation, Université d'Ottawa/University of Ottawa).

Bricout, J., Baker, P. M., Moon, N. W., & Sharma, B. (2021). Exploring the smart future of participation: Community, inclusivity, and people with disabilities. *International Journal of E-Planning Research (IJEPR)., 10*(2), 94–108.

Chemnad, K., & Othman, A. (2024). Digital accessibility in the era of artificial intelligence—Bibliometric analysis and systematic review. *Frontiers in Artificial Intelligence, 7*, 1349668.

Chhimpa, G. R., Kumar, A., Garhwal, S., & Dhiraj. (2024). Empowering individuals with disabilities: a real-time, cost-effective, calibration-free assistive system utilizing eye tracking. *Journal of Real-Time Image Processing, 21*(3), 97.

Collins, A., Rentschler, R., Williams, K., & Azmat, F. (2022). Exploring barriers to social inclusion for disabled people: Perspectives from the performing arts. *Journal of Management & Organization., 28*(2), 308–328.

Dang, B., Ma, D., Li, S., Dong, X., Zang, H., & Ding, R. (2024). Enhancing kitchen independence: Deep learning-based object detection for visually impaired assistance. *Academic Journal of Science and Technology., 9*(2), 180–184.

de Silva, J. D., Pereira, A., Goncalves, R., & Gomes, S. (2014, June 18). State of the art of accessible development for smart devices: From a disable and not impaired point of view. In *2014 9th Iberian Conference on Information Systems and Technologies (CISTI)* (pp. 1–5). IEEE.

Debnath, S., Roy, P., Namasudra, S., & Crespo, R. G. (2023). Retracted article: Audio-visual automatic speech recognition towards education for disabilities. *Journal of Autism and Developmental Disorders., 53*(9), 3581–3594.

Deodhare, D. (2015). *Facial expressions to emotions: A study of computational paradigms for facial emotion recognition* (pp. 173–198). Understanding Facial Expressions in Communication.

Dixon, K., Braye, S., & Gibbons, T. (2022). Still outsiders: The inclusion of disabled children and young people in physical education in England. *Disability & Society., 37*(10), 1549–1567.

Feghali, J. M., Feng, C., Majumdar, A., & Ochieng, W. Y. (2024). Comprehensive review: High-performance positioning systems for navigation and wayfinding for visually impaired people. *Sensors, 24*(21), 7020.

Fosch-Villaronga, E., & Poulsen, A. (2022). Diversity and inclusion in artificial intelligence. *Law and Artificial Intelligence: Regulating AI and Applying AI in Legal Practice*, 109–134.

Furini, M., Gaggi, O., Mirri, S., Montangero, M., Pelle, E., Poggi, F., & Prandi, C. (2022). Digital twins and artificial intelligence: As pillars of personalized learning models. *Communications of the ACM, 65*(4), 98–104.

Ghafoor, K., Ahmad, T., Aslam, M., & Wahla, S. (2024). Improving social interaction of the visually impaired individuals through conversational assistive technology. *International Journal of Intelligent Computing and Cybernetics., 17*(1), 126–142.

Ghulaxe, V. (2024). Robotic process automation with ML and artificial intelligence: Revolutionizing business processes. *International Journal of Engineering Technology and Management Sciences, 4*(8).

Givens, A. R., & Morris, M. R. (2020, January 27). Centering disability perspectives in algorithmic fairness, accountability, & transparency. In *Proceedings of the 2020 conference on fairness, accountability, and transparency* (p. 684).

Hoffman, S. F., & Friedman, H. H. (2018). Machine learning and meaningful careers: Increasing the number of women in STEM. *Journal of Research in Gender Studies, 8*(1).

Hsieh, Y. H., Granlund, M., Odom, S. L., Hwang, A. W., & Hemmingsson, H. (2024). Increasing participation in computer activities using eye-gaze assistive technology for children with complex needs. *Disability and Rehabilitation: Assistive Technology, 19*(2), 492–505.

References

Hughes, C. E., Dieker, L. A., Glavey, E. M., Hines, R. A., Wilkins, I., Ingraham, K., Bukaty, C. A., Ali, K., Shah, S., Murphy, J., & Taylor, M. S. (2022). RAISE: Robotics & AI to improve STEM and social skills for elementary school students. *Frontiers in Virtual Reality, 14*(3), 968312.

Huq, S. M., Maskeliūnas, R., & Damaševičius, R. (2024). Dialogue agents for artificial intelligence-based conversational systems for cognitively disabled: A systematic review. *Disability and Rehabilitation: Assistive Technology, 19*(3), 1059–1078.

Ingavélez-Guerra, P., Robles-Bykbaev, V. E., Perez-Muñoz, A., Hilera-González, J., & Otón-Tortosa, S. (2022). Automatic adaptation of open educational resources: An approach from a multilevel methodology based on students' preferences, educational special needs, artificial intelligence and accessibility metadata. *IEEE Access, 10*, 9703–9716.

Irugalbandara, I. C., Naseem, A. S., Perera, M. S., Logeeshan, V. (2022, June 6). HomeIO: Offline smart home automation system with automatic speech recognition and household power usage tracking. In *2022 IEEE World AI IoT Congress (AIIoT)* (pp. 571–577). IEEE.

Kahlon, Y., Hu, W., Nakatani, M., Maurya, S., Oki, T., Zhu, J., & Fujii, H. (2024). Immersive gaze sharing for enhancing education: An exploration of user experience and future directions. *Computers & Education: X Reality, 5*, 100081.

Karn, A., Singh, P. K., Agarwal, C., Verma, A., Singh, D., & Kumari, M. (2024). Unraveling the power of AI assistants. In *Advances in AI for biomedical instrumentation, electronics and computing* (pp. 473–479). CRC Press.

Kem, D. (2022). Personalised and adaptive learning: Emerging learning platforms in the era of digital and smart learning. *International Journal of Social Science and Human Research, 5*(2), 385–391.

Khalid, U. B., Naeem, M., Stasolla, F., Syed, M. H., Abbas, M., & Coronato, A. (2024). Impact of AI-powered solutions in rehabilitation process: Recent improvements and future trends. *International Journal of General Medicine*, 943–969.

Khamaj, A. (2025). Ai-enhanced chatbot for improving healthcare usability and accessibility for older adults. *Alexandria Engineering Journal, 116*, 202–213.

Khan, M. R. (2024). Role of AI in enhancing accessibility for people with disabilities. *Journal of Artificial Intelligence General Science (JAIGS), 3*(1), 281–291.

Khoury, M. J., Bowen, S., Dotson, W. D., Drzymalla, E., Green, R. F., Goldstein, R., Kolor, K., Liburd, L. C., Sperling, L. S., & Bunnell, R. (2022). Health equity in the implementation of genomics and precision medicine: A public health imperative. *Genetics in Medicine, 24*(8), 1630–1639.

Kumar, A., Nayyar, A., Sachan, R. K., & Jain, R. (Eds.). (2023). *AI-assisted special education for students with exceptional needs*. IGI Global.

Kumar, N., & Jain, A. (2022). A deep learning based model to assist blind people in their navigation. *Journal of Information Technology of Educational Innovation Practice, 21*, 95–114.

Lin, M., Paul, R., Abd, M., Jones, J., Dieujuste, D., Chim, H., & Engeberg, E. D. (2023). Feeling the beat: A smart hand exoskeleton for learning to play musical instruments. *Frontiers in Robotics and AI, 10*, 1212768.

Malcangi, M. (2021). AI-based methods and technologies to develop wearable devices for prosthetics and predictions of degenerative diseases. *Artificial Neural Networks*, 337–354.

Manzoor, S., Iftikhar, S., Ayub, I., Shahid, A., Haq, A. U., Muhammad, W., & Shafique, M. (2024). Range sensor-based assistive technology solutions for people with visual impairment: A review. *Disability and Rehabilitation: Assistive Technology, 19*(3), 576–584.

Mao, C., & Chang, D. (2023). Review of cross-device interaction for facilitating digital transformation in smart home context: A user-centric perspective. *Advanced Engineering Informatics., 57*, 102087.

Mastam, N. M., & Zaharudin, R. (2024). Work readiness skills for students with learning disabilities in special education vocational schools: A conceptual framework. *Jurnal Pendidikan Bitara UPSI, 19*(17), 1.

Megalingam, R. K., Manoharan, S. K., Riju, G., & Mohandas, S. M. (2024, May 17). NETRAVAAD: Interactive eye based communication system for people with speech issues. IEEE Access.

Morina, A., Carballo, R., & Castellano-Beltran, A. (2024). A systematic review of the benefits and challenges of technologies for the learning of university students with disabilities. *Journal of Special Education Technology, 39*(1), 41–50.

Morris, M. R. (2020). AI and accessibility. *Communications of the ACM., 63*(6), 35–37.

Nayak, S., & Das, R. K. (2020, October 7). Application of artificial intelligence (AI) in prosthetic and orthotic rehabilitation. In *Service robotics*. IntechOpen.

Nedjar, I., & M'hamedi, M. (2024). Interactive system based on artificial intelligence and robotic arm to enhance Arabic sign language learning in deaf children. *Education and Information Technologies*, 1–8.

Orynbay, L., Razakhova, B., Peer, P., Meden, B., & Emeršič, Ž. (2024). Recent advances in synthesis and interaction of speech, text, and vision. *Electronics, 13*(9), 1726.

Patthanajitsilp, P., & Chongstitvatana, P. (2022, January 26). Obstacles detection for electric wheelchair with computer vision. In *2022 14th International Conference on Knowledge and Smart Technology (KST)* (pp. 97–101). IEEE.

Phutthammawong, P., Angbunthorn, P., Kaewprapha, P., & Cholaseuk, D. (2020). *Artificial intelligence autonomous vehicle for the blind*.

Piette, J. D., Newman, S., Krein, S. L., Marinec, N., Chen, J., Williams, D. A., Edmond, S. N., Driscoll, M., LaChappelle, K. M., Maly, M., & Kim, H. M. (2022). Artificial Intelligence (AI) to improve chronic pain care: Evidence of AI learning. *Intelligence-Based Medicine, 6*, 100064.

Pydala, B., Kumar, T. P., & Baseer, K. K. (2023). Smart_Eye: A navigation and obstacle detection for visually impaired people through smart app. *Journal of Applied Engineering and Technological Science (JAETS), 4*(2), 992–1011.

Radanliev, P., De Roure, D., Novitzky, P., & Sluganovic, I. (2024). Accessibility and inclusiveness of new information and communication technologies for disabled users and content creators in the Metaverse. *Disability and Rehabilitation: Assistive Technology, 19*(5), 1849–1863.

Regondi, S., Donvito, G., Frontoni, E., Kostovic, M., Minazzi, F., Bratières, S., Filosto, M., & Pugliese, R. (2025). Artificial intelligence empowered voice generation for amyotrophic lateral sclerosis patients. *Scientific Reports, 15*(1), 1361.

Rehan, H. (2023). Shaping the future of education with cloud and AI technologies: Enhancing personalized learning and securing data integrity in the evolving EdTech landscape. *Australian Journal of Machine Learning Research & Applications, 3*(1), 359–395.

Rojas, M., Balderas, D. C., Maldonado, J., Ponce, P., Lopez-Bernal, D., & Molina, A. (2024). Lack of verified inclusive technology for workers with disabilities in industry 4.0: A systematic review. *International Journal of Sustainable Engineering, 17*(1), 1–21.

Sahal, R., Alsamhi, S. H., & Brown, K. N. (2022). Personal digital twin: A close look into the present and a step towards the future of personalised healthcare industry. *Sensors, 22*(15), 5918.

Sahoo, S., & Choudhury, B. (2024). Exploring the use of computer vision in assistive technologies for individuals with disabilities: A review. *Journal of Future Sustainability, 4*(3), 133–148.

Sakthimohan, M., Sakthi, S., Pugalmani, R., Kumar, H., & Rani, E. (2024, March 14). Automated smart home assistive system implementation for physically impaired community using eye gestures. In *2024 10th International Conference on Advanced Computing and Communication Systems (ICACCS)* (Vol. 1, pp. 81–85). IEEE.

Satyavathi, D. M., Rutwik, A., Kumar, N. A., Lokesh, M., Kumar, N. P., & Karthik, P. (2023). AI & IoT enabled smart exoskeleton for rehabilitation of a finger for paralysed people. *Journal of Data Acquisition Process, 38*(2), 4033.

Shahabi, S., Pardhan, S., Shabaninejad, H., Teymourlouy, A. A., Tabrizi, R., & Lankarani, K. B. (2022). Toward good governance for the prosthetics and orthotics sector in Iran: Evidence from a qualitative study. *Prosthetics and Orthotics International, 46*(4), e398-406.

Sharma, P., & Dash, B. (2023). AI and VR enabled modern LMS for students with special needs. *Journal of Foreign Language Education and Technology, 8*(1), 2023.

Siregar, N. C., Gumilar, A., Warsito, W., Amarullah, A., & Rosli, R. (2023). Enhancing STEM learning for all: A paper concept of accessible resources. *Ibn Khaldun International Journal of Applied Sciences and Sustainability, 1*(1), 58–68.

Skowronek, M., Gilberti, R. M., Petro, M., Sancomb, C., Maddern, S., & Jankovic, J. (2022). Inclusive STEAM education in diverse disciplines of sustainable energy and AI. *Energy and AI, 7*, 100124.

Slee, R., & Tait, G. (2022). *Ethics and inclusive education*. Springer.

Souza, L. R., Francisco, R., Tavares, J. E. R., & Barbosa, J. L. (2024). Intelligent environments and assistive technologies for assisting visually impaired people: a systematic literature review. *Universal Access in the Information Society*, 1–28.

Treviranus, J. (2017). Start your machine learning engines and race to the edge! *Transportation Talk*, 14–15.

Trewin, S., Basson, S., Muller, M., Branham, S., Treviranus, J., Gruen, D., Hebert, D., Lyckowski, N., & Manser, E. (2019). Considerations for AI fairness for people with disabilities. *AI Matters, 5*(3), 40–63.

Valipoor, M. M., & De Antonio, A. (2023). Recent trends in computer vision-driven scene understanding for VI/blind users: A systematic mapping. *Universal Access in the Information Society, 22*(3), 983–1005.

Walle, H., De Runz, C., Serres, B., & Venturini, G. (2022). A survey on recent advances in AI and vision-based methods for helping and guiding visually impaired people. *Applied Sciences, 12*(5), 2308.

Wen, L. Y., Morrison, C., Grayson, M., Marques, R. F., Massiceti, D., Longden, C., & Cutrell, E. (2024, May 11). Find my things: Personalized accessibility through teachable AI for people who are blind or low vision. In *Extended Abstracts of the CHI Conference on Human Factors in Computing Systems* (pp. 1–6).

Westley, M., Sutherland, D., & Bunnell, H. T. (2019). Voice banking to support people who use speech-generating devices: New Zealand voice donors' perspectives. *Perspectives of the ASHA Special Interest Groups, 4*(4), 593–600.

Wickramasinghe, N., Ulapane, N., Andargoli, A., Ossai, C., Shuakat, N., Nguyen, T., & Zelcer, J. (2022). Digital twins to enable better precision and personalized dementia care. *JAMIA Open, 5*(3), ooac072.

Wieseler, C. (2022). Disability bioethics, Ashley X, and disability justice for people with cognitive impairments. In *The disability bioethics reader* (pp. 301–312). Routledge.

Yan, Y. (2022). Deep dive into deepfakes—Safeguarding our digital identity. *Brooklyn Journal International of Law, 48*, 767.

Yang, H. F., Ling, Y., Kopca, C., Ricord, S., & Wang, Y. (2022). Cooperative traffic signal assistance system for non-motorized users and disabilities empowered by computer vision and edge artificial intelligence. *Transportation Research Part c: Emerging Technologies, 145*, 103896.

Yang, Q., Jin, W., Zhang, Q., Wei, Y., Guo, Z., Li, X., Yang, Y., Luo, Q., Tian, H., & Ren, T. L. (2023). Mixed-modality speech recognition and interaction using a wearable artificial throat. *Nature Machine Intelligence, 5*(2), 169–180.

Yu, H., Wang, J., Murugesan, M., & Rahman, A. S. (2022). Artificial intelligence-based quality management and detection system for personalized learning. *Journal of Interconnection Networks, 22*(Supp02), 2143004.

Zdravkova, K. (2022, June 16). The potential of artificial intelligence for assistive technology in education. In *Handbook on intelligent techniques in the educational process: Vol 1 recent advances and case studies* (pp. 61–85). Springer International Publishing.

Zdravkova, K., Krasniqi, V., Dalipi, F., & Ferati, M. (2022). Cutting-edge communication and learning assistive technologies for disabled children: An artificial intelligence perspective. *Frontiers in Artificial Intelligence, 5*, 970430.

Chapter 2
The History of AI in Transforming Disability Support

Abstract Disabled individuals have achieved progressive improvements in their daily lives through the advancement of assistive technology throughout the centuries. The evolution of assistive devices from ancient canes and trumpets to the latest AI-powered tools represents the technological advancement of assistance for disabled individuals. The evolution of assistive technology for disabled individuals splits into three distinct eras: the Foundation Period (before 1900) cantered on basic assistance devices followed by the Establishment Period (1900–1972) focused on regulatory frameworks then the Empowerment Period (1973–present) marked the integration of smart assistive technologies from basic machinery to advanced AI-driven digital innovations. This chapter explores the integration of AI technology that has made tremendous advancements in assistive services for disabilities. This chapter explains the historical transformation in assistive technology for disabled individuals from ancient aids to modern AI-based solutions that is from the initial stage of hearing aids and Braille systems and wheelchairs come the latest AI-driven solutions including brain-computer interfaces and computer mobility tools. The chapter reveals the trend toward popular assistive technologies which have become both intelligent and adaptive and personalized through the examination of their advancements. Through this development, AI shapes the way disabled people interact with present-day technology systems.

Keyword Disabled individuals · Ancient aids · Artificial intelligence · Assistive technologies · Independent living

2.1 Introduction

World Health Organization estimates indicate that more than 15% of the global population experiences impairments. Most of these limitations restrict an individual's ability to engage with the outer world overall (World Health Organization, 2022). Currently, the majority of citizens in industrialized nations possess electronic devices,

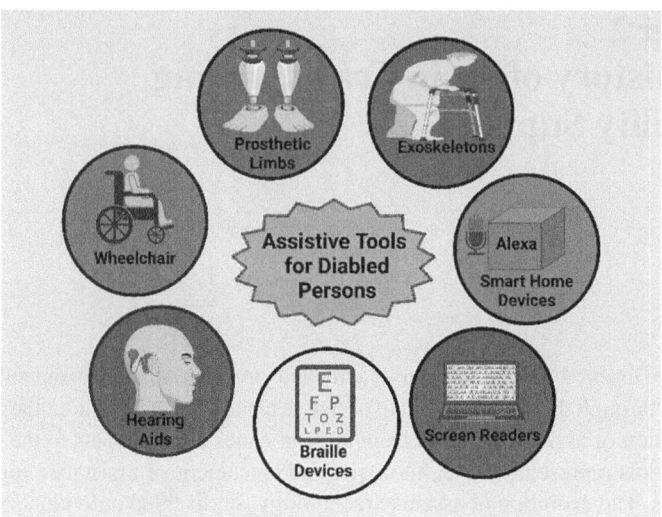

Fig. 2.1 Assistive tools for people with disabilities

such as computers, which they utilize daily to accomplish their activities and objectives efficiently (Firth et al., 2019). Therefore, it is essential to develop appropriate solutions to address the mandatory needs of differently-abled individuals, facilitating their personal and professional lives. Technology has been instrumental in improving individuals' quality of life (Macke et al., 2018). Consequently, an individual requires unrestricted and effortless access to the Internet and technology. There is a necessity to integrate various modifications in assistive technologies via artificial intelligence and computer vision, which can significantly enhance the support for this group (Fig. 2.1).

Physical disabilities encompass disorders such as motor impairment, which includes those afflicted with muscular dystrophy, fractures, or other ailments that result in tremors or diminished fine motor control (Fernandez et al., 2021). These individuals have challenges in performing their daily work. Considering these constraints, this demographic can utilize several AI-based assistive technologies to help them perform various activities (Whittaker et al., 2019). Technology is now more essential than ever to the human experience. Humans engage with various forms of technology daily, ranging from basic tools to intricate systems. In the realm of disability, technology has evolved from a mere instrument for routine activities to a crucial facilitator for attaining autonomy and equity. Accessibility features can be improved with technology, but it's important to remember that people with disabilities have different needs and those needs can change over time (Gregor et al., 2005). People with disabilities may be able to live better lives with the help of technology and mobility. When thinking about these changing and contextual factors, it is important to always pay attention to living experiences and come up with new ideas. Disability, self-perception, and the social stigma associated with technology all influence an individual's expectations.

Assistive technology for disabled people has been around since ancient times when simple tools like walking sticks and hearing horns were used. Technological growth and a growing focus on inclusion led to big steps forward in the twentieth century, such as prosthetics, hearing aids, and mobility devices (Weisman & Dickerson, 2022). When computers came out, they brought with them screen readers and other ways to communicate. The Internet made it easier for people to get jobs and go to school. In the past few years, AI has changed assistive technology by making solutions more specialized and smarter. AI-driven voice recognition systems assist individuals with speech difficulties in communicating effectively, while computer vision technologies aid blind or visually challenged individuals in navigating their environment (Inbamalar & Sreenidhi, 2024). Wearable tech, like smart glasses and brain-computer connections, makes it easier to move around and be independent. Generative AI models help people learn and be creative in even more ways, breaking down hurdles for people with cognitive disabilities (Feltrero & Osuna-Acedo, 2023). This change shows that people are committed to using technology to make life easier and more open to everyone. This chapter illustrates the history of assistive technology, which has progressed from primitive tools like canes and ear instruments to modern, intricate prosthetics and intelligent technologies that are based on artificial intelligence. This evolution is a testament to the ingenuity and compassion of the human spirit.

2.2 Introduction to Technology

Defining the term "technology" accurately is extremely important. People usually say that technology is the use of information and tools to solve problems or reach goals. It includes any instrument, technique, system, or methodology employed by people to create, manipulate, or govern their environment (Carroll, 2017). This encompasses all innovations, ranging from rudimentary implements such as the wheel or lever to intricate systems like computers and cell phones. Technology fundamentally involves the utilization of tools and methodologies to enhance efficiency, productivity, and capabilities (Brynjolfsson & Hitt, 2000). The Jacquard Loom serves as a prominent historical example of technology, automating the intricate process of pattern weaving through the use of punched cards, a method that subsequently impacted the evolution of early computers (Harlizius-Klück, 2017). Comprehending that advancements in "technology" extend beyond the demand for more intelligent phones, computers, or artificial intelligence (AI) is essential for grasping the significance of "tech" for the disability community.

2.3 The Evolution of Assistive Devices

The history of AT can be categorized into three distinct phases, each significantly contributing to the field's evolution. The account of assistive technology history is founded on the evolution of assistive devices, interventions, disability-specific initiatives and educational institutions, as well as legislation about disabilities. The three periods are designated as the Foundation Period (before 1900), Establishment Period (1900–1972), and Empowerment Period (1973–present).

2.3.1 The Foundation Period (Before 1900)

The Foundation Period denotes the extensive timeframe during which assistive technology (AT) was found, initially investigated, and characterized as a resource to aid those with disabilities in their daily activities (King, 2015). This era encompasses any time before 1900, as there is no definitive event recognized as the discovery of AT. It is widely acknowledged that AT was developed in response to an individual's inclination to "act" following a severe injury (Riemer-Reiss, 1997). Consequently, some form of AT has been implemented throughout history. Cook and Hussey (1995) narrate a fictional account of Borg the Caveman to illustrate the emergence of assistive technology (AT). In this narrative, Borg incurs a severe injury that heals inadequately, leading to a conspicuous limp. To compensate for this limp, Borg constructs a cane that suits him, hence resulting in AT, which emerges from humanity's aspiration to sustain work (Cook & Polgar, 2007). The efforts during this period effectively ensured the survival of individuals with severe injuries. This era marked the commencement of expert analysis on the constraints imposed by disabilities, alongside the formulation of programs aimed at imparting academic and life skills to individuals with cognitive, sensory, and motor impairments. These events and discoveries established the foundation for numerous policies, equipment, and interventions being utilized by and for individuals with disabilities (Kudlick, 2003).

2.3.2 The Establishment Period (1900–1972)

The Establishment Period refers to the timeframe during which disability fields were formally recognized as distinct entities. During this period, new policies, regulations, and litigations constituted substantial advancements for individuals with disabilities, their families, and disability advocates (Wendt & Lloyd, 2011). Substantial progress was achieved in the examination of disability prevention and consequences. Moreover, societal perceptions toward disabilities and the capacities of individuals with disabilities have evolved significantly in a favorable direction. During this period, individuals with disabilities constituted an increasing proportion of the population.

Medical advancements have enabled children to survive diseases and birth complications at a significantly higher rate than in previous eras (Marini, 2011). The advancements, coupled with World War I, World War II, the Korean War, and the Vietnam War, resulted in a new cohort of disabled individuals young, injured veterans individuals need assistance to reintegrate into a postwar community facing these new obstacles (Baker, 2012; Mowery & Rosenberg, 1999). These events catalyzed an emphasis on advancing technology to enhance the functional skills of those with diverse disabilities, as well as on enacting disability-related legislation about work and education. These inventions and legislations collaboratively facilitated individuals in utilizing their functional capabilities to mitigate the impacts of their disability and reintegrate into the workforce in unprecedented numbers. The significant population of motivated individuals with impairments has resulted in an unparalleled surge in the creation of assistive technology that persists to this day. The Establishment Period served as a transitional phase. The onset of the period resembled the Foundation Period, since most efforts were focused on creating products and policies for the deaf and blind (Kudlick, 2003). During this period, inclusivity was not a primary concern. As time advanced, this concept began to evolve, establishing the foundation for the Establishment Period.

2.3.3 The Empowerment Period (After 1973–Present)

The Empowerment Period is designated as such due to the ongoing provision of capability and legal authority to individuals with disabilities, enabling them to pursue their life goals. During this period, an unparalleled volume of legislation concerning disability rights has been enacted. The initiative commenced with the Rehabilitation Act of 1973 and has progressed through educational and assistive technology legislation, including the Individuals with Disabilities Education Act of 1997 and the Technology-Related Assistance for Individuals with Disabilities Act of 1988 (Bryant & Seay, 1998; George, 1999; Lewis et al., 2012). This era witnessed ongoing advancements in assistive technology devices, particularly those related to computers, as it aligned with the Information Age. The year 1973 marks the commencement of the Empowerment Period due to the enactment of the Rehabilitation Act of 1973, seen as the inaugural triumph in the disability rights movement (Lewis et al., 2012).

The Empowerment Period persists, characterized by the ongoing enactment of disability-related legislation and the continuous development of assistive technology devices and methodologies, all designed to assist individuals with disabilities in optimizing their functional skills to achieve their objectives. The "desire to accomplish" has been the impetus for AT development across all three periods (Kusec et al., 2019). It initiated the development of products and equipment to assist individuals with impairments during the Foundation Period. The rising population of individuals with disabilities aspiring to pursue the "Healthy Dream" heightened public awareness of this "desire for achievement" throughout the Establishment Period

(Klein et al., 2001). This identical "desire for achievement" has similarly resulted in governmental acknowledgment of disabilities via legislation designed to assist those with disabilities in "achieving" during the Empowerment Period. The AT field has a significant history and a promising future grounded in the principles of advocacy and the inclusion of individuals with disabilities in all settings.

2.4 Evolution of Assistive Devices

Assistive technology (AT) encompasses any equipment, instrument, program, or system that enhances, sustains, or improves the functional capabilities of individuals with impairments (Scherer, 2011). This technology can range from a basic cardboard communication board to intricate devices such as tailored prosthetics, switches, screen readers, hearing aids, wheelchairs, adaptive scissors, or advanced software, among numerous more instances (Fig. 2.1) (Wong, 2020).

The history of AT development is extensive and always evolving. Upon close examination, a consistent pattern emerges in technological advancements. Frequently, innovations developed for disability assistance subsequently extend their use to mainstream applications. This underscores the universal advantage of including accessibility in design, an approach that benefits those with disabilities while simultaneously improving technology usability for all users (Marini, 2011). The history of assistive technology exemplifies resilience, ingenuity, and compassion. What began with basic aids has transformed into a varied spectrum of technologies that enable individuals with disabilities to achieve greater independence and engage comprehensively in society (Lewis et al., 2012). As technology advances, chances to improve the quality of life for individuals of all abilities will also increase.

Ramps and curb cuts designed for wheelchair accessibility also serve as an efficient option for strollers, shopping carts, rolling baggage, and similar items (Aldoukhi et al., 2023). Closed captioning was originally developed for the deaf and hearing-impaired community and now also benefits individuals who require audio to be muted in public or quiet environments, as well as assisting non-native speakers of a language. The same applies to audiobooks, automatic door openers, and electric toothbrushes. Assistive technology transcends mere tools; it aims to dismantle obstacles, broaden opportunities, and guarantee that all individuals, irrespective of their ability, can flourish and contribute to a more promising future (Holloway & Barbareschi, 2022). The following section explains the evolution of assistive technology for disabled individuals.

2.4.1 Ancient Roots of Assistive Technology

The origins of assistive technology can be traced to ancient cultures. The origins of assistive technology for individuals with disabilities can be traced back to ancient civilizations, where rudimentary tools and devices were crafted to aid mobility and functionality. In Egypt and Greece, people who had trouble walking used simple tools like canes to help them. The first examples include simple crutches and canes made from wood to help people having trouble moving around. At the same time, people in Rome and Egypt started making simple prosthetic arms out of metal and wood to replace lost limbs (Bourrier, 2020). An ancient Egyptian wooden toe is an example of a prosthetic limb that shows the way people with physical disabilities first tried to improve their usefulness and sense of dignity (Sigounas, 2023). In a similar vein, the Greeks and Romans developed wheelchairs and wagons to improve mobility, indicating a recognition of the importance of specialized aids (Bulliet, 2016). Many of these old tools were made with materials and skills that were common in the area. This demonstrates the proficiency of early communities in addressing physical challenges. Along with movement aids, the first hearing aids were simple gadgets that used hollowed-out horns or shells to boost sound (Bulliet, 2016). Historical records show that people tried to teach sign language and other ways to communicate, which shows that people were aware of the needs of people with sensory problems (Joseph, 2020). Even though these tools didn't have the most advanced features of modern technologies, they paved the way for the creation of helpful devices. People came up with these innovations because they wanted to improve their quality of life and make it easier for them to take part in social and business activities (Baynton, 1996). By dealing with the problems that people with disabilities faced, ancient societies set the stage for acceptance and flexibility. When people first realized they needed help with everyday tasks, it led to innovations that are still changing people's lives today, showing a long-lasting commitment to removing barriers and promoting freedom (Voss, 2024).

2.4.2 Communication Advancement by Braille

When Braille was invented, it was a big step forward as helpful technology that made it easier for blind people or have low vision to communicate. When Louis Braille invented Braille in 1824, it was a big step forward in the field of helpful technology. This tactile writing system, which was developed by Louis Braille in 1824, was designed to address the deficiencies of previous methods for communication among the blind, such as raised letters, which were both ineffective and burdensome. Louis lost his sight as a child and came up with the Braille system, which is a way to write by touching and using raised dots to show letters and numbers (Oliphant, 2008). Inspired by a military code called "night writing" Braille, a French teen who went blind young in life came up with a method using six raised dots arranged in a rectangle. Touch-based reading and writing work well because each set of dots stands for a letter, number, or sign. Braille is a global tool for education and self-sufficiency because it is easy to use and can be used for languages, music notation, and math. This invention made it possible for blind people to read and write on their own, which had a huge impact on their ability to learn and communicate (Jiménez et al., 2009).

Braille initially encountered opposition from educators and institutions; however, its efficacy and the advocacy of its users ultimately led to its broad acceptance. When schools for the blind started using the system in the late 1800s, they did so because they knew it could help people learn and interact on their own. Braille's invention changed education by giving blind people access to reading, writing, and intellectual growth. It is still an important tool for empowering people. In the digital era, innovations like refreshable Braille displays and electronic Braille writers have increased accessibility (Longmore et al., 2001). Louis Braille's innovative creation transformed communication and represented the persistent human effort to foster innovation and dismantle barriers, promoting inclusion and equality for individuals with disabilities.

2.4.3 Evolution of Hearing Aids

The development of hearing aids represents a significant advancement in assistive technology for people with hearing impairments, facilitating increased inclusivity and enhancing quality of life. The first attempts to help people having trouble hearing used tools like ear tubes, which picked up sound and sent it into the ear (Mills, 2009). In the past, hearing aids were simple tools like ear trumpets and acoustic horns from the seventeenth century that made sounds louder for people having trouble hearing. Despite their limited functionality and frequent cumbersomeness, these passive tools offered the first practicable method for individuals with hearing disabilities to participate more actively in social settings and conversations.

The twentieth century brought about big changes, like the first electrically amplified hearing aids that used carbon mics and later ones that used vacuum tube technology. In the twentieth century, the first electric hearing aids were made. These were big machines that used vacuum tubes to boost sound (Uchanski & Sarli, 2019). Even though the initial electrical models were quite large and of limited utility, they represented a significant advancement in the ability of individuals with hearing impairments to become more cognizant of their surroundings. The 1950s brought the transistor, allowing for the creation of smaller and more effective hearing aids. This marked an exciting advancement in technology for those with hearing difficulties. During the 1950s, advancements in transistor technology paved the way for the development of smaller and more dependable devices, such as behind-the-ear (BTE) models. These models simplified the process of obtaining hearing aids and rendered them more discrete (Schillmeier et al., 2022).

Individuals with hearing difficulties have experienced many changes in their lives since the digital transformation of the late twentieth century. Digital signal processing (DSP) allows for customized sound amplification that meets individual hearing requirements, all while minimizing background noise and enhancing speech clarity (Nisha et al., 2022). Bluetooth connectivity, smartphone control, and artificial intelligence are some of the more advanced features in modern hearing aids that make it easy for users to switch between sound options (Lawenrence et al., 2024).

These enhancements not only aid in restoring hearing but also empower individuals with hearing disabilities to engage in school, work, and social activities, fostering independence and societal acceptance.

2.4.4 From Wheelchairs to Advanced Mobility Aids

Wheelchairs have a rich history that stretches back for centuries. Straightforward wheelchair designs have been discovered in China and Greece. Beginning with basic wheelchairs and advancing to more sophisticated mobility devices demonstrate significant strides in addressing the needs of individuals with physical disabilities. Mobility aids such as wooden sticks and basic wheelchairs have existed since ancient times, providing valuable support for those facing challenges in movement. The first self-propelled wheelchair, created in the 1600 s, offered individuals a new sense of independence and marked a significant milestone in the evolution of assistive devices (Meiklejohn-Kerr, 2024). Even so, the initial designs were difficult to navigate and had restricted capabilities, leading many to seek assistance.

Before the twentieth century, significant advancements were absent. The twentieth century introduced fresh ideas and changes as people became more aware of disabilities and the significance of including everyone. In the mid-twentieth century, mobility aids evolved with the introduction of lightweight materials and powered alternatives. These changes helped people with physical challenges navigate more easily and enjoy greater freedom. Wheelchairs were once crafted from heavy steel or wood, but today they are designed with lighter materials such as aluminum (Ko, 2022). This allows for easier movement and usage. When electric bicycles emerged in the mid-twentieth century, people transformed their modes of transportation. They could easily move around on their own now. These devices featured electric motors and key controls, allowing individuals with limited upper body strength to move around with ease.

Nowadays, mobility aids have evolved to offer a variety of options for different needs. Adjustable bicycles and robotic exoskeletons exemplify the advancements in technology. These tools help disabled people move around more easily and feel more independent and secure. Smart wheelchairs equipped with sensors, GPS, and voice control provide improved navigation and safety features (Leaman & La, 2017). These improvements show a move toward creating gadgets that are easy for everyone to use, allowing people with disabilities to fully take part in society. This underscores that innovation may eliminate barriers and foster equity.

2.4.5 Communication by Computer Accessibility

The arrival of computers provided new choices for people with disabilities. Computer accessibility has transformed communication for those with disabilities, eliminating barriers and enabling their participation in a connected digital environment (Kravchenko et al., 2022). People with physical, sensory, or cognitive disabilities often face major difficulties when using regular computer systems. New assistive technologies have turned computers into valuable resources for freedom, learning, and social connection. Screen readers, developed in the 1970s and 1980s, help visually impaired users read digital material by converting text into speech or Braille. Early tools like screen readers and magnifiers were created for people with vision problems. They turned text on a screen into spoken words or made the text bigger (Soto, 2020). Speech recognition software lets people with mobility challenges use their voices to handle computers and type, giving them more independence. Verbal instructions have enabled individuals with limited mobility to operate computers and devices as a result of advancements in speech recognition technology (Juang & Rabiner, 2005).

Accessibility for those with severe physical limitations has been further enhanced with the emergence of alternative input devices such as eye-tracking systems, switch-based controllers, and adaptable keyboards (Khaleel et al., 2023). These tools allow people with restricted movement to use digital systems effectively. For people having hearing difficulties, real-time captions and text-to-speech help make online material easier to understand.

Modern advancements have integrated artificial intelligence and machine learning into accessibility solutions. AI-powered tools, such as predictive text and natural language processing, simplify communication for individuals with cognitive or speech impairments (ElHennawy, 2024). Innovations like haptic feedback and gesture recognition enhance accessibility for users with diverse needs. Moreover, the rise of inclusive design ensures that accessibility is built into mainstream technology rather than being an afterthought. By removing barriers to digital interaction, computer accessibility has opened doors to education, employment, and social inclusion for millions of people with disabilities, fostering empowerment and equality in the digital age (Harpur, 2013).

2.4.6 Smart Modern Innovative Devices

Currently, assistive technology is advancing swiftly. Modern innovations in smart devices, powered by artificial intelligence (AI), have revolutionized the lives of individuals with disabilities, offering unparalleled autonomy, accessibility, and inclusion as compared to conventional assistive tools (Fig. 2.2) (Almufareh et al., 2024). Smartphones and tablets provide accessibility features such as screen magnification, voice control, and text-to-speech functionalities, facilitating daily chores for

2.4 Evolution of Assistive Devices

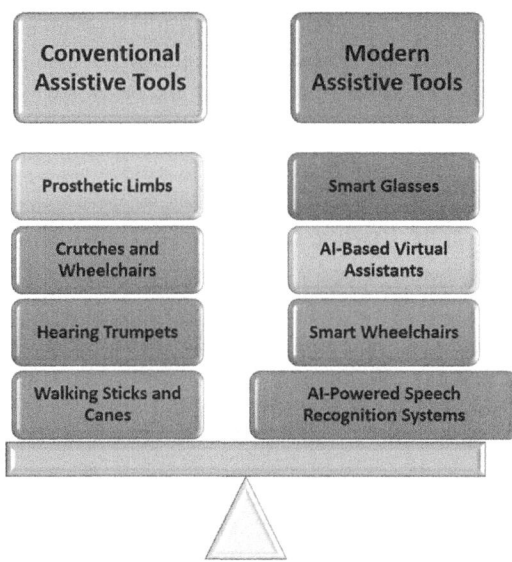

Fig. 2.2 Comparison between convention and modern assistance tools for people with disabilities

individuals with disabilities. AI-driven technologies such as virtual assistants—like Amazon Alexa, Google Assistant, and Apple's Siri—enable the hands-free operation of smart home devices, allowing individuals with mobility impairments to control lighting, appliances, and even security systems through simple voice commands. These devices reduce dependence on caregivers, enhancing independence in daily living (Esquivel et al., 2024).

For sensory impairments, AI has bridged critical gaps in communication and interaction. Smart hearing aids with AI-powered noise cancellation adapt to different sound environments, improving clarity and reducing strain for individuals with hearing disabilities (Lawenrence et al., 2024). Speech-to-text and real-time captioning apps, fueled by AI algorithms, allow seamless communication for the deaf or hard of hearing. Similarly, AI-driven tools like Microsoft's Seeing AI app and envision smart glasses provide real-time object identification, text reading, and navigation assistance for individuals with visual impairments, significantly enhancing their ability to navigate the world independently (Nasser et al., 2024).

AI's integration into advanced mobility aids, such as smart wheelchairs and prosthetics, has been transformative. AI-enabled prosthetics employ machine learning to replicate natural movements, providing users with increased control and comfort, while smart wheelchairs are equipped with AI-based navigation systems that identify obstacles and recommend the most efficient routes (Nayak & Das, 2020). Prosthetics have improved a lot, with many models now using robots and artificial intelligence to move like natural limbs. Brain-computer interfaces (BCIs) allow individuals with severe disabilities to operate computers and communicate solely using their brain signals, utilizing artificial intelligence (Awuah et al., 2024). These AI-driven innovations not only enhance accessibility but also promote inclusivity, allowing individuals with disabilities to fully engage in social life, employment, and education, while simultaneously redefining the potential of assistive technology.

2.5 The Future of Assistive Technology

Significant advancements in assistive technology are anticipated in the future. New technologies like brain-computer interfaces (BCIs) can connect the brain directly to devices, offering new chances for people with significant disabilities. AI offers advantages for people with disabilities (Fig. 2.3).

2.5.1 AI Enhancing Accessibility by Assistive Technology

Assistive technology powered by AI plays a crucial role in promoting the rights specified in the Convention on the Rights of Persons with Disabilities (Winzer & Mazurek, 2017). AI technology can empower individuals facing challenges to experience greater independence and engage more fully in society. Ensuring broad access to these technologies is essential for meeting the commitments made by states under the CRPD, promoting inclusivity and accessibility in healthcare (Smith & Smith, 2024). Assistive technology powered by AI provides solutions that enhance mobility, communication, and everyday tasks, bridging the divide between ability and access.

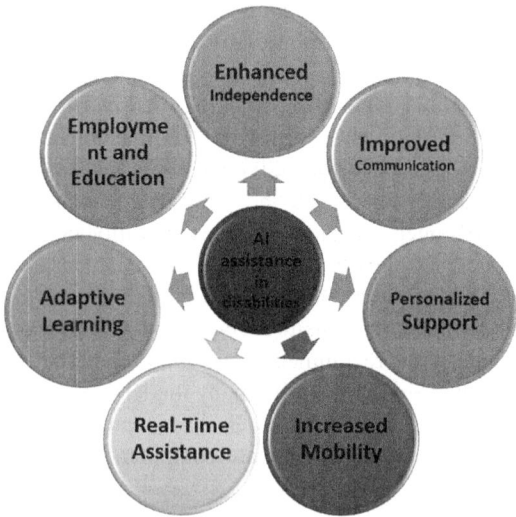

Fig. 2.3 Advantage of AI assistance for people with disabilities

Many other types of assistive technologies can leverage artificial intelligence to improve themselves. Smart wheels and communication tools designed for those with speech difficulties are two such. By enabling impaired persons to engage in activities they might not be able to perform prior, these tools can significantly enhance their quality of life. For instance, artificial intelligence smart wheelchairs can help users negotiate their surroundings by identifying obstacles and creating best paths (Pancholi et al., 2024). Individuals with speech difficulties can more effectively articulate their thoughts by utilizing tools that incorporate natural language processing. In various spheres, including education, employment, and social events, these technologies not only grant impaired individuals more freedom but also facilitate their participation in society.

2.5.2 Daily Living Assistance

AI-driven solutions are transforming the assistance available to those with disabilities in their daily tasks. Artificial intelligence (AI) has become a major force in improving the quality of life and freedom of disabled people by providing personalized, intuitive, and highly effective solutions that help them do daily tasks. Smart home assistance that can be controlled by voice can help disabled people get their daily tasks done more quickly (Mtshali & Khubisa, 2019). Voice commands let people having trouble moving control smart home devices, set reminders, and do things like manage their plans or make calls through AI-powered virtual assistants like Amazon Alexa, Google Assistant, and Apple Siri. These tools can control lighting, appliances, and many other systems in the home, making it easier for people to go about their daily lives. These hands-free exchanges make people less reliant on caregivers and give them more control over their daily lives (Jabbar et al., 2019). Smart home assistants can also send notifications and reminders, which can help people stay organized and take care of their health and fitness. For sensory disabilities, AI provides groundbreaking tools to navigate and interact with the environment. Applications like Microsoft's Seeing AI and Google Lookout leverage computer vision to describe objects, people, and text in real time for visually impaired users. Similarly, AI-driven captioning tools, such as Otter.ai and Ava, provide real-time transcriptions for individuals with hearing impairments, enabling seamless communication in social and professional settings (Mrayhi et al., 2024).

Mobility aids integrated with AI have also revolutionized personal assistance. Smart wheelchairs equipped with AI-based navigation systems can identify obstacles and suggest optimal paths, while wearable exoskeletons help users with mobility impairments regain physical movement (Muthu et al., 2023). Brain-computer interfaces (BCIs), powered by AI, allow individuals with severe disabilities to operate devices, communicate, and even control prosthetics using brain signals. Innovations like mind-controlled exoskeletons and intelligent house assistants promote independent living. These technologies boost accessibility and promote inclusivity, allowing individuals with disabilities to lead more independent lives (Almufareh et al., 2024).

Mind-controlled exoskeletons enable users to execute movements and tasks with enhanced efficiency, while smart home assistants facilitate the operation of numerous household gadgets via voice commands or alternative interfaces, thereby rendering daily activities more manageable. A major development in assistive technology, mind-controlled exoskeletons let people with mobility problems take control over their body motions. These systems use brain-computer interfaces to convert neurological impulses into commands that run the exoskeleton, therefore allowing users to do tasks that would be either difficult or impossible otherwise (Memon, 2024). Apart from its utility, AI technologies offer tailored help and adaptive learning fit to the particular needs of every person. By adding artificial intelligence into assistive devices, society is moving toward a time when disabilities will not limit involvement in daily life, therefore fostering more inclusivity and equality.

2.5.3 BCI Techniques Advancing Assistive Technologies

AI techniques have produced a range of helpful technologies including brain-computer interfaces and smart wheelchairs. With these technologies, people with physical restrictions may be more independent and productive (Pancholi et al., 2024). Nevertheless, issues still need to be resolved before these technologies may be generally applied. While brain-computer interfaces let individuals run equipment through cognitive commands, intelligent wheelchairs are able to navigate autonomously. Constant research and development help to guarantee that these technologies benefit a wider audience by raising their dependability, accuracy, and economy of cost. Cutting-edge technology called brain-computer interfaces, or BCIs, allow individuals to use their brainwaves to control electronics (He et al., 2020). For those with severe physical restrictions, this can be especially beneficial since it provides a fresh approach of interacting with their surroundings (Khuntia & Manivannan, 2023). More studies are required to make BCIs more precise and dependable while also reducing their cost and degree of difficulty so that more individuals might utilize them. AI-equipped intelligent wheelchairs enable users to move about on their own, therefore facilitating more safe and efficient mobility. These wheelchairs use sensors and machine learning systems to locate impediments, create paths, and modify their speed and direction as needed. Still, these systems must always be developed to ensure they can manage several situations and user requirements.

2.6 Conclusion

Helpful technological advances demonstrate an enthusiastic spirit to simplify tasks for disabled individuals as well as improve their social inclusion. The assistive development from early aids to smart devices along with AI-powered prosthetics has improved quality of life for people with disabilities. Assistive tools have proven crucial for creating an independent society by removing barriers so all people can feel welcomed. The development of AI-based assistance provides new possibilities for rehabilitation tools that adapt to individuals along with smart support systems. Innovative help systems created through AI combine the advantages of contemporary technology with designs suitable for all people to increase disability autonomy. This development brings both independence and fair treatment into daily activities. For assistive technology to get better, AI needs to come up with solutions that make them quicker and easier for everyone to use. The world will achieve a better standard of living through independent existence for all people.

References

Aldoukhi, M., Angel, M., Bare, L., Blacher, D., Cawi, J., Chabanel, T., Ciccone, M., Clapper, K., El Jai, S., Ferrer, A., & Figueroa, P. (2023). *Access of persons with disabilities to public ground transportation and roadways.*

Almufareh, M. F., Kausar, S., Humayun, M., & Tehsin, S. (2024). A conceptual model for inclusive technology: Advancing disability inclusion through artificial intelligence. *Journal of Disability Research, 3*(1), 20230060.

Awuah, W. A., Ahluwalia, A., Darko, K., Sanker, V., Tan, J. K., Pearl, T. O., Ben-Jaafar, A., Ranganathan, S., Aderinto, N., Mehta, A., & Shah, M. H. (2024, May 22). *Bridging minds and machines: the recent advances of brain-computer interfaces in neurological and neurosurgical applications.* World Neurosurgery.

Baker, M. S. (2012). Military medical advances resulting from the conflict in Korea, Part I: Systems advances that enhanced patient survival. *Military Medicine, 177*(4), 423–429.

Baynton, D. C. (1996). *Forbidden signs: American culture and the campaign against sign language.* University of Chicago Press.

Bourrier, K. (2020). Mobility impairment. A cultural history of disability in the long nineteenth century, *5*, 43

Bryant, B. R., & Seay, P. C. (1998). The technology-related assistance to individuals with disabilities act: Relevance to individuals with learning disabilities and their advocates. *Journal of Learning Disabilities, 31*(1), 4–15.

Brynjolfsson, E., & Hitt, L. M. (2000). Beyond computation: Information technology, organizational transformation and business performance. *Journal of Economic Perspectives, 14*(4), 23–48.

Bulliet, R. W. (2016, December 31). *The wheel: Inventions and reinventions.* Columbia University Press.

Carroll, L. S. (2017). A comprehensive definition of technology from an ethological perspective. *Social Sciences, 6*(4), 126.

Cook, A. M., & Polgar, J. M. (2007, October 1). *Cook and Hussey's assistive technologies-e-book.* Elsevier Health Sciences.

ElHennawy, S. M. (2024). The impact of artificial intelligence (AI) in the assessment and treatment of communication disorders (a review of literature). *The Egyptian Journal of Language Engineering, 11*(2), 36–45.

Esquivel, P., Gill, K., Goldberg, M., Sundaram, S. A., Morris, L., & Ding, D. (2024). Voice assistant utilization among the disability community for independent living: A rapid review of recent evidence. *Human Behavior and Emerging Technologies, 1*, 6494944.

Feltrero, R., & Osuna-Acedo, S. (2023, November 26). Social innovation on educational AI developments. A case study on social participation on designing AI generative models for diversity. In *International Symposium on Emerging Technologies for Education* (pp. 16–26). Springer Nature Singapore.

Fernandez, H. H., Walter, B. L., Rush, T., & Ahmed, A. (Eds.). (2021, August 4). *A practical approach to movement disorders: Diagnosis and management.* Springer Publishing Company.

Firth, J., Torous, J., Stubbs, B., Firth, J. A., Steiner, G. Z., Smith, L., Alvarez-Jimenez, M., Gleeson, J., Vancampfort, D., Armitage, C. J., & Sarris, J. (2019). The, "online brain": How the Internet may be changing our cognition. *World Psychiatry, 18*(2), 119–129.

George, M. C. (1999). A new idea: The individuals with disabilities education act after the 1997 amendments. *Law & Psychological Review, 23*, 91.

Gregor, P., Sloan, D., & Newell, A. F. (2005). Disability and technology: Building barriers or creating opportunities? *Advances in Computers, 64*, 283–346.

Harlizius-Klück, E. (2017). Weaving as binary art and the algebra of patterns. *Textile, 15*(2), 176–197.

Harpur, P. (2013). From universal exclusion to universal equality: Regulating ableism in a digital age. *Northern Kentucky Law Review, 40*, 529.

He, B., Yuan, H., Meng, J., & Gao, S. (2020). Brain–computer interfaces. *Neural Engineering*, 131–183.

Holloway, C., & Barbareschi, G. (2022, May 31). *Disability interactions: creating inclusive innovations.* Springer Nature.

Inbamalar, T. M., & Sreenidhi, K. (2024, April 4). Artificial intelligence powered eye for visually challenged people. In *2024 Ninth International Conference on Science Technology Engineering and Mathematics (ICONSTEM)* (pp. 1–5). IEEE.

Jabbar, W. A., Kian, T. K., Ramli, R. M., Zubir, S. N., Zamrizaman, N. S., Balfaqih, M., Shepelev, V., & Alharbi, S. (2019). Design and fabrication of smart home with internet of things enabled automation system. *IEEE Access, 23*(7), 144059–144074.

Jiménez, J., Olea, J., Torres, J., Alonso, I., Harder, D., & Fischer, K. (2009). Biography of louis braille and invention of the braille alphabet. *Survey of Ophthalmology, 54*(1), 142–149.

Joseph, F. (2020, August 4). *Ancient high tech: The astonishing scientific achievements of early civilizations.* Simon and Schuster.

Juang, B. H., & Rabiner, L. R. (2005, January 1). Automatic speech recognition—A brief history of the technology development. *Georgia Institute of Technology. Atlanta Rutgers University and the University of California, 67*, 1.

Khaleel, A. H., Abbas, T. H., & Abdul-Wahab, S. I. (2023). Enhancing Human-Computer Interaction: A Comprehensive Analysis of Assistive Virtual Keyboard Technologies. *Ingenierie des Systemes D'information, 28*(6), 1709.

Khuntia, P. K., & Manivannan, P. V. (2023). Review of neural interfaces: Means for establishing brain-machine communication. *SN Computer Science, 4*(5), 672.

King, S. (2015). Constructing the disabled child in England, 1800–18601. *Family & Community History, 18*(2), 104–121.

Klein, S., & Schive, K. (Eds.). (2001, April 1). *You will dream new dreams: Inspiring personal stories by parents of children with disabilities.* Kensington Books.

Ko, H. Y. (2022, May 18). Wheelchairs and wheelchair mobility in spinal cord injuries. In *Management and rehabilitation of spinal cord injuries* (pp. 837–860). Springer Nature Singapore.

Kravchenko, O., Koliada, N., Berezivska, L., Dikhtyarenko, S., Baida, S., & Danylevych, L. (2022). Digital barrier-free and psychosocial support for students with disabilities in distance learning environments. *International Journal of Computer Science & Network Security, 22*(8), 15–24.

Kudlick, C. J. (2003). Disability history: Why we need another "other." *The American Historical Review, 108*(3), 763–793.

Kusec, A., Velikonja, D., DeMatteo, C., & Harris, J. E. (2019). Motivation in rehabilitation and acquired brain injury: Can theory help us understand it? *Disability and Rehabilitation, 41*(19), 2343–2349.

Lawenrence, E., Chakraborty, S., & Dudekula, C. S. (2024). Smart earphones. In *Handbook of artificial intelligence and wearables* (pp. 246–260). CRC Press.

References

Leaman, J., & La, H. M. (2017). A comprehensive review of smart wheelchairs: Past, present, and future. *IEEE Transactions on Human-Machine Systems, 47*(4), 486–499.

Lewis, A. N., Cooper, R. A., Seelman, K. D., Cooper, R., & Schein, R. M. (2012). Assistive technology in rehabilitation: Improving impact through policy. *Rehabilitation Research, Policy & Education, 26*(1).

Longmore, P. K., & Umansky, L. (Eds.). (2001). *The new disability history: American perspectives.* NYU Press.

Macke, J., Casagrande, R. M., Sarate, J. A., & Silva, K. A. (2018). Smart city and quality of life: Citizens' perception in a Brazilian case study. *Journal of Cleaner Production., 182*, 717–726.

Marini, I. (2011, July 27). The history of treatment toward persons with disabilities. In I. Marini, N. M. Glover-Graf, & J. Millington (Eds.). *Psychosocial aspects of disability: Insider perspectives and counseling strategies.*

Meiklejohn-Kerr, H. (2024). From ancient adaptations to modern innovations: A historical perspective of disability inclusive furniture. *Humanities Journal, 1*(3), 2024011.

Memon, Q. A. (2024). A comprehensive review of current assistive technology research for paralyzed people. *Current and Future Trends on Intelligent Technology Adoption, 2*, 287–305.

Mills, M. (2009). When mobile communication technologies were new. *Endeavour, 33*(4), 141–147.

Mowery, D. C., & Rosenberg, N. (1999, October 28). *Paths of innovation: Technological change in 20th-century America.* Cambridge University Press.

Mrayhi, S., Khribi, M. K., Belhadj, H., & Jemni, M. (2024). Designing future education for all: Principles and frameworks. In *Envisioning the future of education through design* (pp. 147–177). Springer Nature Singapore.

Mtshali, P., & Khubisa F. (2019, March 6). A smart home appliance control system for physically disabled people. In *2019 Conference on Information Communications Technology and Society (ICTAS)* (pp. 1–5). IEEE.

Muthu, P., Tan, Y., Latha, S., Dhanalakshmi, S., Lai, K. W., & Wu, X. (2023). Discernment on assistive technology for the care and support requirements of older adults and differently-abled individuals. *Frontiers in Public Health, 10*, 1030656.

Nasser, N., Ali, A. Y., Karim, L., & Al-Helali A. (2024, April 9). *Enhancing mobility for the visually impaired with AI and IoT-enabled mobile applications.* ScienceOpen Preprints.

Nayak, S., & Das, R. K. (2020, October 7). Application of artificial intelligence (AI) in prosthetic and orthotic rehabilitation. In *Service robotics.* IntechOpen.

Nisha, K. V., Devi, N., & Sridhar, S. (2022, September 23). Music to ears in hearing impaired: Signal processing advancements in hearing amplification devices. In *Advances in speech and music technology: Computational aspects and applications* (pp. 217–236). Springer International Publishing.

Oliphant, J. (2008). "Touching the light": The invention of literacy for the blind. *Paedagogica Historica, 44*(1–2), 67–82.

Pancholi, S., Wachs, J. P., & Duerstock, B. S. (2024). Use of artificial intelligence techniques to assist individuals with physical disabilities. *Annual Review of Biomedical Engineering, 26.*

Riemer-Reiss, M. L. (1997). *Factors associated with assistive technology discontinuance among individuals with disabilities.* University of Northern Colorado.

Scherer, M. J. (2011, December 20). *Assistive technologies and other supports for people with brain impairment.* Springer Publishing Company.

Schillmeier, M., Stock, R., & Ochsner, B. (Eds.). (2022). *Techniques of hearing: History, theory and practices.* Taylor & Francis.

Sigounas, V. (2023). *Prosthetic entanglements: Living with transnational prosthetic limb design in Uganda and the United States.* Doctoral dissertation, The University of North Carolina at Chapel Hill.

Smith, L., & Smith, P. (2024). The ethical issues raised by the use of Artificial Intelligence products for the disabled: An analysis by two disabled people. In *Ethics in online AI-based systems* (pp. 121–134). Academic Press.

Soto, M. Á. (2020). *Interactive tactile representations to support document accessibility for people with visual impairments*, Doctoral dissertation, Universität Stuttgart.

Uchanski, R. M., & Sarli, C. C. (2019). 20th century hearing devices: Going, going nearly gone. *The Hearing Journal, 72*(12), 10–12.

Voss, A. (2024, November 8). *The future we're building: How today's innovations will shape tomorrow's world*. eBookIt.com.

Weisman, G., & Dickerson, G. (2022, November 15). *History of rehabilitation engineering*. In *Rehabilitation Engineering* (pp. 3–44). CRC Press.

Wendt, O., & Lloyd, L. L. (2011, January 1). Definitions, history, and legal aspects of assistive technology. In *Assistive technology: Principles and applications for communication disorders and special education* (pp. 1–22). Brill.

Whittaker, M., Alper, M., Bennett, C. L., Hendren, S., Kaziunas, L., Mills, M., Morris, M. R., Rankin, J., Rogers, E., Salas, M., & West, S. M. (2019, November 8). *Disability, bias, and AI*. AI Now Institute.

Winzer, M., & Mazurek, K. (2017, March 17). The convention on the rights of persons with disabilities: Reconstructing disability to reimagine education. In *The Wiley handbook of diversity in special education* (pp. 1–22).

Wong, G. (2020). The role of assistive technology in enhancing disability arts. *Review of Disability Studies: An International Journal, 16*(1), 1–31.

World Health Organization. (2024, July 31). *Universal health coverage partnership annual report 2022: More than 10 years of experiences to orient health systems towards primary health care*. World Health Organization.

Chapter 3
Empowering Disabled People with AI

Abstract Artificial intelligence has the capacity to substantially augment the capabilities of individuals with disabilities by improving accessibility, autonomy, and overall quality of life. The use of AI-driven technologies is revolutionizing disability support, diminishing obstacles, and promoting inclusivity. Innovations such as enhanced communication devices for individuals with speech impairments and AI-driven help for the visually impaired, hearing impaired, and physically crippled are transforming the way individuals confront everyday obstacles. AI-driven robotics, intelligent wheelchairs, and rehabilitation technologies are transforming mobility and personal support, while AI-based educational tools are fostering more inclusive learning environments. AI enhances accuracy, promotes seamless communication, and personalizes support systems, thereby bridging gaps and fostering more fair opportunities for those with impairments. This chapter examines the various methods by which AI empowers individuals with disabilities, illustrating the way intelligent technologies improve communication, mobility, rehabilitation, and education, thereby promoting a more inclusive and accessible society for everyone.

Keyword Disability support · Visual assistance · Cognitive disability · Advanced technology · Robotics

3.1 Introduction

Devices or algorithms capable of performing cognitive tasks typically executed by humans are referred to as artificial intelligence (AI) (Korteling et al., 2021). This includes several technical methods that aim to replicate human behavior and address problems with reasoning analogous to that employed in chess. A subclass of artificial intelligence, machine learning allows algorithms exposed to more data to learn and improve their performance to forecast individual demand (Sarker, 2021). Google uses machine learning, for example; its algorithms compile information on users' social network interests and search queries to provide more customized search results and recommendations. The Google search engine is used by around 4 billion people worldwide; hence, artificial intelligence is considered as a social advantage. Everyone has access, including those with limitations. Improving accessibility depends much on technology, particularly artificial intelligence (Chemnad & Othman, 2024). Prioritizing solutions that enhance the quality of life for a certain group overcomes the pursuit of the latest developments. For about a billion people with disabilities worldwide could use artificial intelligence, this marks major progress.

For handicapped people, artificial intelligence can greatly improve access. Image recognition (Fernando et al., 2025), facial recognition (Zhao et al., 2018), lipreading recognition (Ivanko et al., 2019), text summarization (Alarcon et al., 2024), and real-time captioning or translation (Kawas et al., 2016) are some methods to address accessibility challenges. It can also assist individuals with hearing problems, cognitive challenges, and visual impairments. For people with impairments, artificial intelligence greatly affects their daily lives; for example, a person with a cognitive disability could easily understand their surroundings by means of text summarizing. What initially appears to be a complex message to interpret ultimately reveals itself as a comprehensible text. Daily, actions that were formerly difficult or unattainable are now readily accessible. Through the utilization of AI, individuals with disabilities can navigate surroundings that recognize and address their issues (Zhang & Tao, 2020). As time goes on, technology makes it easier to access artificial intelligence, which in turn helps to make the world a more inclusive place. By putting all people regardless of constraints on an equal basis, artificial intelligence promotes equality.

3.2 AI Benefits for Disability Support

AI accessibility has various facets, one of which involves utilizing AI to assist those with disabilities (Fig. 3.1). The subsequent section elucidates the manner in which AI enables their autonomy.

3.2.1 Communication

AI-enabled communication technologies have revolutionized the way individuals with disabilities connect with others, breaking barriers to interaction and fostering inclusivity. Numerous applications employ artificial intelligence to enhance accessibility. These advanced systems employ state-of-the-art capabilities such as natural language processing, speech recognition, and machine learning to enhance conversational fluency (Vinothkumar & Karunamurthy, 2023). Communication with others can be challenging, contingent upon the type of disability and individual characteristics. For individuals with speech impairments, devices equipped with AI-powered text-to-speech converters offer a voice, allowing them to express their thoughts and feelings. Similarly, speech-to-text systems help those with hearing impairments by providing real-time transcription of spoken words (Orynbay et al., 2024).

3.2 AI Benefits for Disability Support

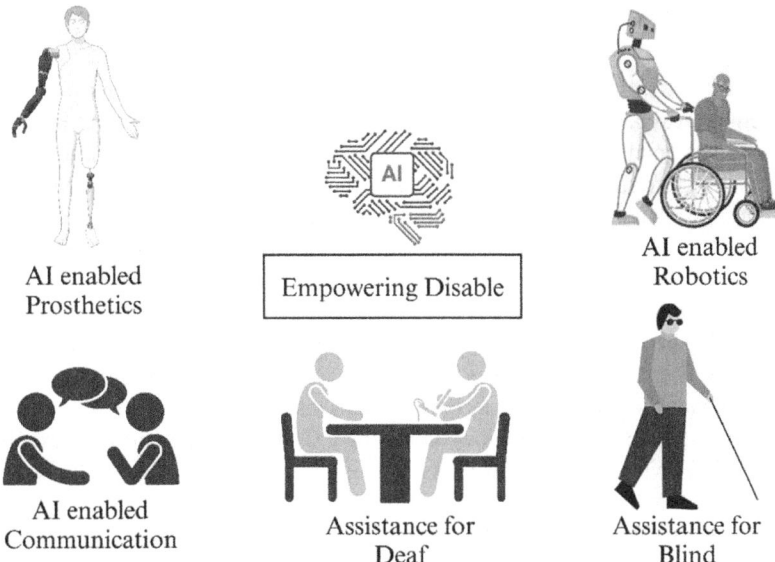

Fig. 3.1 AI accessibility tools assisting disabled

However, technology and AI ensure inclusivity and can serve individuals with disabilities. Wearable artificial intelligence (AI)-driven gadgets like smart glasses translate text into voice or offer navigational aid, therefore empowering those with visual disabilities (Almufareh et al., 2024). Enhanced with artificial intelligence, augmentative and alternative communication (AAC) devices provide predictive text and context-aware recommendations, therefore simplifying the communication process for people with motor disabilities (Pitt & Ousley, 2024). Beyond personal contacts, artificial intelligence helps impaired people in social and professional settings using automatic subtitles, gesture recognition, and emotion detection, thus facilitating virtual attendance at conferences and events.

Moreover, by using quick translating tools and encouraging cross-cultural relationships, artificial intelligence helps the disabled worldwide connectedness by breaking language boundaries. Maintaining relationships with others in a culture going more and more digital might be difficult for disabled people that rely on the Internet and social media and have growing importance. Improved using artificial intelligence algorithms, social media channels offer tailored content and accessibility choices so that handicapped people may interact with communities all around and share their experiences (Packin, 2021). These developments not only close gaps in communication but also increase self-expression, independence, and social integration. AI-enabled communication tools show the transforming power of invention in building a society more inclusive, linked, and sympathetic for all people, regardless of ability.

3.2.2 Assistance for the Visually Impaired

AI-enabled technologies have revolutionized communication for blind or visually impaired individuals, enhancing their independence and connectivity. Tools like screen readers and text-to-speech systems convert digital content into audio, making it accessible (Fitria, 2022). Many uses of artificial intelligence are under development currently that assist blind or visually challenged people in communication. For instance, "VoiceOver" is a screen reader directly included in cell phones. VoiceOver uses artificial intelligence to define app icons, and battery status, and partially describe images even though it mostly uses it to articulate emails or text messages (Smaradottir et al., 2018). The Android equivalent of VoiceOver is referred to as TalkBack. Users can fully utilize their cell phones (Tomlinson et al., 2016). Presenting Siri, the virtual assistant for iPhones. Voice control makes it simple for users to communicate, whether they are texting a friend or conducting a Google search. Siri is an excellent tool for anyone with visual impairments to maintain communication with their loved ones (Abdolrahmani et al., 2018). Windows includes Microsoft's virtual assistant, Cortana. It facilitates computer navigation for individuals with visual impairments and blindness by enabling the exclusive use of voice commands. The system is fairly analogous to Siri (Sharma et al., 2020). An application named Google Assistant can be activated by voice commands. Users may effortlessly configure an alarm or organize their schedule, like Siri. Additionally, AI-powered smart glasses describe surroundings, identify objects, and read text aloud, while navigation apps with GPS and AI provide audio-guided assistance through complex environments (Satani et al., 2020). Furthermore, Braille display devices and handwriting-to-audio converters further aid communication (Lee et al., 2004). Social media platforms and digital interfaces are increasingly designed with accessibility in mind, fostering inclusivity. These innovations empower visually impaired individuals to engage meaningfully in personal, professional, and social interactions, creating a more inclusive society.

3.2.3 Assistance for Deaf People

AI-enabled technologies have transformed communication for deaf or hard-of-hearing individuals, fostering inclusivity and independence (Alkahtani, 2024). Real-time speech-to-text systems, such as live transcription apps, convert spoken language into text, allowing seamless participation in conversations. For example, "Ava" is an instantaneous transcribing application that employs artificial intelligence to transcribe group conversations in real time. The algorithm incorporates punctuation, the speaker's name, and requisite language from the user's lexicon (Selvi et al., 2024). This is a simple method enabling individuals with hearing impairments to participate in conversations with multiple persons without lipreading. Additionally, AI-powered video conferencing platforms now offer automatic captions, enabling accessibility in virtual meetings and events. For example, "RogerVoice" is a French application for fast transcription of group talks, supporting 90 languages. It operates identically to Ava (Sridhar et al., 2023). Sign language recognition tools, powered by AI, translate gestures into text or speech, bridging communication gaps. Additionally, wearable devices provide visual or vibrational alerts for auditory cues like alarms or doorbells (Premsai & Thiyagu, 2024). These advancements empower deaf individuals to connect effectively in personal, professional, and social settings, ensuring a more inclusive and accessible society.

3.2.4 Assistance for Physically Disabled

AI-enabled technologies have greatly enhanced communication and connectivity for individuals with physical disabilities, promoting independence and inclusion. Adaptive devices powered by AI, such as eye-tracking systems and voice-controlled interfaces, enable users with limited mobility to operate computers, smartphones, and other devices seamlessly (Ntoa et al., 2022). Individuals with mobility impairments can utilize virtual assistants like Siri, Google Assistant, and Google Voice Access to operate their phones vocally (Tulshan & Dhage, 2018). Individuals with restricted dexterity constituted the primary target demographic for Google Voice Access. IFTTT is an application that incorporates many apps, enabling users with limited dexterity to utilize all the capabilities of their smartphones with ease (Mineraud et al., 2016). To perform tasks like sending a tweet or vocalizing an email, it creates combinations with programs. Advanced speech recognition tools allow hands-free typing and control, while predictive text and smart suggestions simplify interactions. For instance, using AI technology with the Voiceitt app helps those with speech problems. Individuals with neurological problems, such as Parkinson's disease or brain injuries, may exhibit speech that is initially difficult to understand; nevertheless, Voiceitt uses machine learning to interpret it effectively (Balgude et al., 2024). This tool enables individuals with speech impairments to speak clearly and understandably by standardizing speech for audio or text outputs. Certainly, AI applications and smartphones are not the sole means for those with impairments to communicate and engage with others. Guaranteeing equitable access and services for all individuals, irrespective of their disabilities, is an ongoing objective of online accessibility initiatives (Lewthwaite, 2014).

Designing an accessible website is undoubtedly challenging; yet, AI technology proves to be transformative. The design of a site must be examined and evaluated through machine learning. It can thereafter enhance its accessibility through various avenues like AI software for facial recognition to substitute CAPTCHAs, which can provide challenges for individuals with visual impairments. It is possible to improve usability and navigation for those with mobility disabilities by changing the keyboard's 'Tab' key's function or location (Spalteholz, 2012). Using sounds and gestures, a voice recognition or speech recognition system like Google's Project Euphonia helps people with speech problems use the Internet (Cave, 2024). Additionally, wearable technologies equipped with AI assist in performing everyday tasks, such as operating appliances or navigating environments. AI-enabled audio descriptions for individuals with visual impairments empower the disabled. Web videos can be translated and captioned for people with hearing loss using programs like Microsoft Translator (Millett, 2021). Accessibility for individuals with visual impairments can be significantly enhanced through the modification of graphic components, including typography, color schemes, and spacing. A comprehensive repository of slang, idioms, and phrases that are atypically employed for those with cognitive impairments (Balkom, 2022). Machine learning emulates a browser, akin to its simulation of human behavior, to autonomously adjust screen content and enhance accessibility for individuals with disabilities. Artificial intelligence technology significantly improves accessibility and inclusivity. Robotics and prosthetics, integrated with AI, further enhance mobility and functionality (Nayak & Das, 2020). Consequently, individuals with physical limitations can more effectively engage in all facets of life, encompassing personal relationships, professional endeavors, and social interactions.

3.3 Conversational Systems for Cognitive Disabilities

AI-powered conversational agents have shown promising outcomes for individuals with cognitive impairments, including Parkinson's disease and dementia (Huq et al., 2024). For older and intellectually challenged people, these technologies can improve cognitive assistance and communication, therefore enhancing their quality of life. It is imperative to build conversational bots with different qualities meant for people with cognitive problems (Pancholi et al., 2024). Ensuring effective communication and support involves creating simple interfaces, tailored responses, and robust error-handling systems. The personalizing of conversational artificial intelligence systems is a noteworthy success in this field. By employing machine learning techniques, these systems may learn from user interactions and modify their responses accordingly. This level of personalization is crucial for those with cognitive limitations who may require particular types of engagement and assistance to connect with AI systems. An intuitive interface is crucial for ensuring these technologies are accessible to everybody, even individuals with less technical proficiency (Willingham et al., 2024). For those with cognitive problems, simple and easy interfaces help to lower the learning curve and improve usability. Good error-handling skills are crucial since they let the artificial intelligence effectively control miscommunications or misunderstandings, thereby guaranteeing flawless and encouraging user involvement.

3.4 Inclusive Design in Conversational AI

Achieving health equity in healthcare settings depends on inclusive chatbots being developed and implemented. Patients, AI developers, and healthcare professionals must collaborate within a comprehensive framework to ensure the inclusive advancement of conversational AI systems (Nadarzynski et al., 2024). Ensuring that AI tools meet the many needs of people with disabilities, promoting equal access to healthcare services, and so lowering prejudices that may otherwise impede their usefulness and scope depend on this inclusive approach. Inclusive design calls for the awareness of the several challenges people with disabilities might encounter across interacting with artificial intelligence systems (Smith & Smith, 2021). This includes limits in the areas of the body, senses, cognition, and emotions. Conversational agents utilize advanced natural language processing (NLP) models to understand user inputs and reply appropriately, although these models necessitate continuous adjustment to meet the needs of diverse users (Bansal et al., 2024). For the chatbot to customize its responses according to the user's emotional or situational context, natural language processing algorithms could enhance their effectiveness through sentiment analysis and intent recognition. Individuals requiring comprehensive explanations or step-by-step instructions would appreciate the system's capacity for advanced discourse facilitated by its multi-turn dialogue capabilities.

To comprehend these challenges and devise effective solutions, developers must involve individuals with disabilities in the design process. Accessibility for individuals with diverse disabilities can be attained through the use of many interaction modalities, such as text, speech, and visual aids. Examples of such multimodal solutions include accessible voice-activated interfaces for the visually handicapped and simplified text-based interfaces for those with cognitive problems (Jaddoh et al., 2024). Integrating real-time language translation into chatbots enhances their accessibility for non-native speakers and multilingual organizations. To confirm their practical relevance, these features have to be rigorously tested in actual settings. A more inclusive user experience depends on the chatbot's understanding and reaction to various communication styles and preferences being facilitated. Moreover, constant user comments and testing are crucial for spotting and fixing any flaws that can arise during the actual application. Continuous enhancement is assured by evaluation employing criteria such as customer satisfaction scores, task completion rates, and the chatbot's proficiency in addressing various inquiries. To ensure chatbots remain responsive to the evolving needs of users, collaboration with disability advocacy organizations for ongoing feedback is essential.

3.5 Advanced Robotics for Physical Assistance

AI-powered robots have become essential assistants for those with mobility impairments. These robots are generally accepted for their capacity to foster autonomy and independence; however, concerns regarding their functionality and design persist (Sørensen et al., 2024). Maximizing the efficacy and user acceptability of robotic assistance depends on its being tailored to specific needs. This means adjusting the features of the robots to carry out specific tasks requested by users, therefore guaranteeing simplicity of use and minimizing any psychological barriers to their acceptance. Basic tasks such as object retrieval fall within the robotic assistant's capabilities, while more complex duties like personal care assistance are within their area of proficiency. Various ordinary activities, like eating, drinking, and dressing, can be facilitated with robotic arms. Exoskeletons equipped with advanced sensors provide powered help for ambulation and standing, thereby aiding patients with restricted mobility. This facilitates improved physical rehabilitation and diminishes dependence on caretakers (Rodríguez-Fernández et al., 2021). Robots can adjust to their environment and users' requirements with machine learning algorithms that facilitate predictive control and real-time motion monitoring.

These robots' design and utility have to be carefully assessed to ensure their effectiveness and simplicity for use. It is imperative to implement safety measures, such as obstacle detection sensors and fail-safe algorithms, to prevent accidents during operation. Furthermore, ensuring the robots' adaptability to several surroundings such as congested homes or crowded public spaces helps to increase their utilization. Ergonomic designs enhance the accessibility of straightforward user interfaces, such as wearable controllers and touch screens, for individuals with various mobility impairments. To promote the adoption and extensive utilization of robotic assistants, it is essential to confront psychological barriers such as concerns regarding privacy and the potential reduction of human interaction. One method to establish customer trust is to involve them in the co-design of robotic functionalities. Another approach is to provide customization choices, such as customized voice assistants or adaptive learning elements that align with individual preferences. Working together with disability advocacy groups and medical professionals will help to guarantee that these systems satisfy the particular needs of people with disabilities. Evaluating user acceptance via usability testing and trust indices provides critical insights for improving robotic designs and functioning (Olawade et al., 2025).

3.6 Smart Wheelchair Mobility

The ability of robotics to improve user safety and autonomy is demonstrated by the development of wheelchair mobility devices boosted by artificial intelligence. The development of power wheelchair driving assistance modules enables users to practice navigation and surmount obstacles in simulated environments. These developments underscore the necessity of collaboration to address the complex needs of individuals with disabilities through AI. Such systems can include adaptive speed control, path planning, and obstacle recognition and avoidance to provide safe and effective mobility. Those with limited physical ability notably benefit from this.

AI-enabled wheelchairs significantly enhance users' mobility and independence through superior navigation and control capabilities (Kumar et al., 2024). Algorithms for route planning identify optimal paths, while obstacle detection systems aid users in circumventing obstructions. Moreover, variable speed control guarantees a safe and enjoyable experience by changing the wheelchair's pace depending on the user's preferences and surroundings. Wheelchair operation user training can be facilitated by virtual surroundings, therefore improving confidence and driving skills. Users can engage in practice and learning inside a safe environment by simulating real-world scenarios in these virtual realms.

3.7 Smart Technologies for Rehabilitation and Exercise

For people with impairments, creative technology including virtual reality, wearable devices, and telecommunication tools is improving rehabilitation and exercise possibilities. Combining these technologies with artificial intelligence will help to overcome barriers to physical activity involvement, hence addressing health inequities (Willingham et al., 2024). Customized rehabilitation programs made possible by artificial intelligence improve their efficacy and accessibility by means of their inclusion. Wearable devices can track progress in real time, virtual reality can replicate therapeutic settings, and healthcare providers and patients can engage remotely through telecommunication networks.

Immersive and interactive environments are provided by virtual reality technology, which improves the engagement and enjoyment of rehabilitation exercises. Through the simulation of real-world settings, virtual reality enables users to refine and enhance their physical skills within a secure and regulated environment (Yang et al., 2022). By tracking users' progress and adjusting the complexity of exercises to fit their current capacity, artificial intelligence algorithms can help to ensure that rehabilitation programs remain both demanding and effective. Wearable devices—such as smart clothing and fitness trackers—may continuously track users' physical activity and provide instantaneous feedback. This information guarantees that workouts are tailored to individual demands and capacities, hence personalizing rehabilitation regimens (Sumner et al., 2023). Furthermore, remote monitoring and assistance made possible by communications systems let medical professionals evaluate the development and provide direction without requiring in-person interactions.

3.8 Assistance in Education for Disabled Students

Generative AI is providing innovative solutions that address the specific learning demands of impaired students, thereby transforming education and enhancing accessibility. By leveraging advanced algorithms, generative AI creates personalized learning experiences, adapting content to suit the capabilities of students with disabilities (Fig. 3.2) (Addy et al., 2023). For example, visually impaired students benefit from AI-generated audio descriptions of visual content, while students with hearing impairments gain access to real-time captions and sign language translations for lectures and discussions. Researchers have hypothesized that students with disabilities may greatly benefit from using generative AI in their coursework due to the many obvious advantages it offers, such as, in reading, generative AI can help students with disabilities understand complicated ideas by summarizing and identifying important topics in papers (Tamdjidi, 2023). For writing, when teachers aren't accessible, generative AI services can step in as individualized writing instructors (McCarthy & Yan, 2024). Thirdly, AI can assist with proofreading, which includes fixing spelling and grammar mistakes. Also in class, students with disabilities may be able to engage more completely if generative AI is used to help them develop their communication skills through the provision of discussion topics and other tools (Botchu et al., 2024).

Generative AI also supports students with learning disabilities by generating simplified explanations, interactive lessons, and engaging visual aids tailored to their

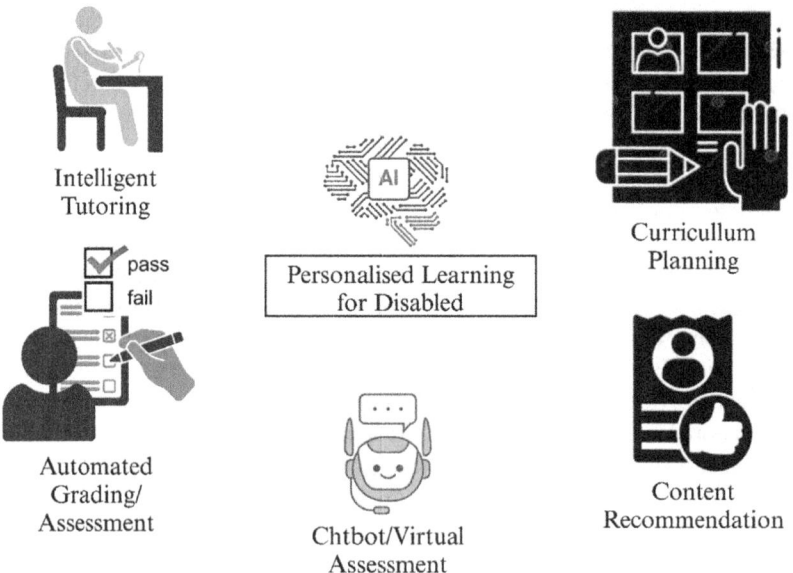

Fig. 3.2 AI-based personalized learning for students with disabilities

cognitive needs. Tools for text-to-speech and speech-to-text enable flawless communication and information intake, therefore enabling students with physical limitations to engage meaningfully in academic environments (McCarthy & Yan, 2024). AI-driven chatbots and virtual tutors provide round-the-clock assistance, clarifying doubts and reinforcing concepts in a personalized manner. Indirectly, generative AI can help kids with disabilities by raising the bar for classroom instruction. For instance, it can verify if the material is accessible. In particular, it has the potential to be taught to recognize the first symptoms of learning difficulties (Johnson et al., 2023), which would allow teachers to develop individualized lesson plans for kids with disabilities (Bozkurt et al., 2023). Generative artificial intelligence presents a more inclusive and encouraging learning environment using both direct and indirect advantages (Chen & Zhu, 2023). This means that students with disabilities will have better access to educational materials, which could lead to better learning outcomes. Moreover, generative AI fosters creativity and collaboration by enabling disabled students to create essays, art, or music using AI tools, leveling the playing field for self-expression. An inclusive and equitable educational environment is achievable since generative AI offers innovative solutions to accessibility challenges, enabling students with disabilities to thrive academically and socially (Michel-Villarreal et al., 2023).

3.9 Empower Independent Living

AI-enabled technologies have revolutionized independent living for individuals with disabilities, empowering them to lead more autonomous and fulfilling lives. These advancements leverage artificial intelligence to address diverse needs, from mobility and communication to daily living tasks and healthcare. AI technology pertains to various domains and can consequently improve accessibility inside the home environment. Through voice commands or mobile apps, smart home systems driven by artificial intelligence let people manage lights, appliances, and security, so increasing the accessibility of homes (Venkatraman et al., 2021). For all people with disabilities, virtual assistants can improve their quality of life. Smart speakers, like the Amazon Echo with Alexa or the Google Home with Google Assistant, enable those with disabilities to manage various home appliances with voice commands, encompassing lighting, alarm scheduling, and music playback (Vlahos, 2019). The capability to connect any household device enables individuals without sight to run their oven using Alexa's voice, while those with limited dexterity can modify room temperature with vocal commands. Individuals with impairments can manage their home virtual assistants remotely using the IFTTT application, even before reaching home. Commonly known as "applets" it incorporates several applications, including virtual assistants like Alexa (Cobb et al., 2020). Individuals with restricted dexterity will find it advantageous, since they may utilize their voices for control, enabling the device to perform any function autonomously. For example, some people turn up the thermostat on their way home.

For those with physical disabilities, AI-driven robotic assistants and wearable devices provide critical support in performing tasks such as cooking, cleaning, and personal care. AI-enabled navigation systems, including GPS apps and smart wearables, help visually impaired individuals navigate urban environments safely and confidently (Nasser et al., 2024). A linked smart home can actually save lives; for example, if someone with disabilities falls, a pre-configured system can call emergency personnel. Because of this, people with disabilities can live on their own with the knowledge that they will be protected in the case of an accident. Likewise, text-to-speech and speech-to-text technologies facilitate natural communication for individuals with speech or hearing disabilities (Orynbay et al., 2024). AI-powered gadgets monitor vital signs, remind users to take their meds, and notify caregivers in case of an emergency so guaranteeing better health management and safety in the field of healthcare. For those with physical limitations, prostheses combined with artificial intelligence change to fit their movements, therefore increasing mobility and freedom (Almufareh et al., 2024).

By providing tools like adaptable learning platforms, easily available work interfaces, and virtual collaborative spaces catered to different needs, artificial intelligence also advances inclusivity in employment and education (Almufareh et al., 2024). Platforms driven by artificial intelligence can enable disabled people to socialize and enjoy entertainment, therefore promoting a feeling of involvement and belonging. AI-enabled technologies facilitate independent living for individuals with impairments, enhancing their quality of life and ensuring their full participation in society through the elimination of barriers and the development of tailored solutions (Araujo-Filho & do Rêgo, 2024). In the end, technological solutions based on artificial intelligence allow individuals with impairments to achieve greater independence and comfort in their own homes. Accessibility is substantially enhanced by artificial intelligence.

3.10 Equal Access to Services

By bridging major accessibility gaps, AI-enabled technologies have empowered persons with disabilities to access the same services as everyone else, therefore promoting equality and inclusion. These developments use artificial intelligence to eliminate obstacles in public areas, healthcare, transportation, and education. For example, AI-powered screen readers and voice assistants enable visually impaired individuals to navigate websites, use apps, and access digital services effortlessly (Brotosaputro et al., 2024). Speech-to-text and real-time captioning systems provide deaf individuals with equal access to educational content, virtual meetings, and entertainment platforms. Inclusivity signifies that all individuals have the right to access services irrespective of their characteristics and impairments. Individuals with visual impairments can read using Braille, while those with hearing impairments may understand films via subtitles. For example, Braille AI Tutor is a novel remedy to address the deficiency of Braille instructors (Srivastava et al., 2021). AI-driven speech recognition and gamification enable blind pupils to acquire Braille skills with greater

3.10 Equal Access to Services

autonomy. Education becomes an essential right. Blind people cannot acquire work or reach social inclusion without access to education. Also, people with impairments can still access the information from the document they need, due to tools like Adobe Accessibility Checker and Microsoft Accessibility Checker (Carter & Markel, 2015).

In healthcare, AI-driven telemedicine platforms offer personalized and accessible consultations, while wearable devices monitor health conditions and alert caregivers when needed (Boppana, 2022). With the use of AI and robot-assisted technologies, the medical field can achieve more precision during surgery and improve the accuracy of diagnoses through data collecting. This is a significant advancement in enhancing the quality of life for individuals with impairments. The creation of an artificial intelligence (AI) exoskeleton that rehabilitates mobility in paraplegic individuals is the most notable example (Nayak & Das, 2020). The development of a technological and medical innovation is beneficial to individuals with motor impairments.

Public transportation systems enhanced with AI provide audio-visual cues and real-time updates, making travel more convenient for individuals with physical or sensory impairments (Soliman et al., 2023). Smart kiosks and automated systems in banks, government offices, and retail spaces use AI to offer user-friendly interfaces, ensuring disabled individuals can perform tasks independently (Mamun et al., 2024). For example, Seeing AI for iOS is an application tailored for individuals with visual impairments, capable of reading and describing various documents positioned beneath the smartphone camera, including banknotes and correspondence. It can distinguish images, colors, and faces, so offering insights into individuals' emotions. The counterpart of Seeing AI is Lookout for Android. Its Quick Scan Mode allows one to quickly review a text (Borgström & Luengprakarn, 2023).

Furthermore, AI-based translation tools, including sign language recognition and gesture-based interfaces, bridge communication gaps, enabling seamless interaction in diverse settings. These advancements guarantee that people with impairments can participate fully in education, work, and social life, accessing the same services as their peers. For example, Google's Project Guideline is an AI-driven system that empowers visually impaired individuals to run independently (Deriba et al., 2024). Equipped solely with a strap around their waist, an Android smartphone attached, and headphones, visually impaired individuals can run independently according to a guideline marked on the ground (Manzoor et al., 2024).

Several more solutions exist and are being developed by startups and huge organizations like Google and Microsoft that utilize AI to improve the lives of individuals with disabilities in various industries. To improve accessibility, AI technologies take a user-centered approach, which means they utilize inclusive design to think of ways to help individuals with impairments. AI technology enhances their daily independence by rendering the world more accessible and inclusive, whether they are at home seeing a subtitled film or at work engaging with an accessible document. By addressing diverse needs with innovative solutions, AI fosters inclusivity, dismantles barriers, and creates a world where equal access to services is a standard for all.

3.11 Conclusion

AI technologies possess the capacity to significantly improve the lives of those with impairments in multiple areas. Through a user-centered methodology, AI-driven solutions utilize inclusive design to address the specific requirements of impaired individuals, enhancing accessibility and promoting increased independence. Technologies such as subtitles for the hearing impaired, screen readers for the visually impaired, and AI-driven assistive devices enhance the seamlessness and inclusivity of daily activities. Artificial intelligence significantly contributes to workplaces by facilitating knowledge access via adaptive tools, hence promoting equitable possibilities for all individuals. Furthermore, innovations in robotics and customized rehabilitation technology are transforming mobility and assistance services. By tackling the various obstacles encountered by those with disabilities, AI fosters a more egalitarian and accessible society. Through ongoing improvement, AI possesses the significant potential to revolutionize disability support, enabling individuals to achieve greater independence and fulfillment in their lives.

References

Abdolrahmani, A., Kuber, R., & Branham, S. M. (2018, October 8). "Siri Talks at You" an empirical investigation of voice-activated personal assistant (VAPA) usage by individuals who are blind. In *Proceedings of the 20th international ACM SIGACCESS conference on computers and accessibility* (pp. 249–258).

Addy, T., Kang, T., Laquintano, T., & Dietrich, V. (2023). Who benefits and who is excluded?: Transformative learning, equity, and generative artificial intelligence. *Journal of Transformative Learning, 10*(2), 92–103.

Alarcon, R., Moreno, L., Martínez, P., & Macías, J. A. (2024). EASIER system. Evaluating a Spanish lexical simplification proposal with people with cognitive impairments. *International Journal of Human–Computer Interaction, 40*(5), 1195–1209.

Alkahtani, B. N. (2024). The impact of artificial intelligence on quality of life for deaf and hard of hearing students. *American Annals of the Deaf, 169*(4), 329–347.

Almufareh, M. F., Kausar, S., Humayun, M., & Tehsin, S. (2024). A conceptual model for inclusive technology: Advancing disability inclusion through artificial intelligence. *Journal of Disability Research, 3*(1), 20230060.

Araujo-Filho, I., & do Rêgo, A. C. (2024). Leveraging artificial intelligence to enhance the quality of life for patients with autism spectrum disorder: A comprehensive review. *Journal of Surgical and Clinical Research, 15*(2), 141–172.

Balgude, S. D., Gite, S., Pradhan, B., & Lee, C. W. (2024). Artificial intelligence and machine learning approaches in cerebral palsy diagnosis, prognosis, and management: A comprehensive review. *Peer Journal of Computer Science, 10*, e2505.

Bansal, G., Chamola, V., Hussain, A., Guizani, M., & Niyato, D. (2024). Transforming conversations with AI—A comprehensive study of ChatGPT. *Cognitive Computation*, 1–24.

Boppana, V. R. (2022). Impact of telemedicine platforms on patient care outcomes. *Innovative Engineering Sciences Journal, 2*(1).

Borgström, L., & Luengprakarn, T. (2023). *Designing accessible medical information: Understanding the challenges and opportunities for blind and visually impaired individuals.*

References

Botchu, B., Iyengar, K. P., & Botchu, R. (2024). Can ChatGPT empower people with dyslexia? *Disability and Rehabilitation: Assistive Technology, 19*(5), 2131–2132.

Bozkurt, A., Junhong, X., Lambert, S., Pazurek, A., Crompton, H., Koseoglu, S., Farrow, R., Bond, M., Nerantzi, C., Honeychurch, S., & Bali, M. (2023). Speculative futures on ChatGPT and generative artificial intelligence (AI): A collective reflection from the educational landscape. *Asian Journal of Distance Education, 18*(1), 53–130.

Brotosaputro, G., Supriyadi, A., & Jones, M. (2024). AI-powered assistive technologies for improved accessibility. *International Transactions on Artificial Intelligence, 3*(1), 76–84.

Carter, J., & Markel, M. (2015). Web accessibility for people with disabilities: An introduction for web developers. *Writing and Speaking in the Technology Professions: A Practical Guide, 1*, 484–492.

Cave, R. (2024). *How people living with motor neurone disease use personalised automatic speech recognition technology to support social interaction.* Doctoral dissertation, UCL (University College London).

Chemnad, K., & Othman, A. (2024). Digital accessibility in the era of artificial intelligence—Bibliometric analysis and systematic review. *Frontiers in Artificial Intelligence, 7*, 1349668.

Chen, B., & Zhu, X. (2023). Integrating generative AI in knowledge building. *Computers and Education: Artificial Intelligence., 5*, 100184.

Cobb, C., Surbatovich, M., Kawakami, A., Sharif, M., Bauer, L., Das, A., & Jia, L. (2020). How risky are real users' {IFTTT} applets?. In *Sixteenth Symposium on Usable Privacy and Security (SOUPS 2020)* (pp. 505–529).

Deriba, F. G., Wubineh, B. Z., & Teka, M. Z. (2024, November 18). Review of AI technologies for enhancing the lives of visually impaired individuals: Applications, outcomes, and future directions. In *2024 International Conference on Information and Communication Technology for Development for Africa (ICT4DA)* (pp. 241–246). IEEE.

Fernando, S., Ndukwe, C., Virdee, B., & Djemai, R. (2025). Image recognition tools for blind and visually impaired users: An emphasis on the design considerations. *ACM Transactions on Accessible Computing, 18*(1), 1–21.

Fitria, T. N. (2022). Utilizing text-to-speech technology: Natural reader in teaching pronunciation. *JETLEE: Journal of English Language Teaching, Linguistics, and Literature, 2*(2), 70–78.

Huq, S. M., Maskeliūnas, R., & Damaševičius, R. (2024). Dialogue agents for artificial intelligence-based conversational systems for cognitively disabled: A systematic review. *Disability and Rehabilitation: Assistive Technology, 19*(3), 1059–1078.

Ivanko, D., Ryumin, D., & Karpov, A. (2019). Automatic lip-reading of hearing impaired people. *The International Archives of the Photogrammetry, Remote Sensing and Spatial Information Sciences, 42*, 97–101.

Jaddoh, A., Loizides, F., Rana, O., & Syed, Y. A. (2024). Interacting with smart virtual assistants for individuals with dysarthria: A comparative study on usability and user preferences. *Applied Sciences, 14*(4), 1409.

Johnson, C., Smart, K., & Mahar, P. (2023) Is there a place for generative artificial intelligence in special education? *National Social Science Technology Journal, 48*.

Kawas, S., Karalis, G., Wen, T., & Ladner, R. E. (2016, October 23). Improving real-time captioning experiences for deaf and hard of hearing students. In *Proceedings of the 18th International ACM SIGACCESS Conference on Computers and Accessibility* (pp. 15–23).

Korteling, J. H., van de Boer-Visschedijk, G. C., Blankendaal, R. A., Boonekamp, R. C., & Eikelboom, A. R. (2021). Human-versus artificial intelligence. *Frontiers in Artificial Intelligence, 4*, 622364.

Kumar, A., Singh, M., Singh, M., Ramprabu, J., Dubey, A., & Mujoo, S. (2024). A novel electronic wheel chair design using artificial intelligence assisted smart sensors and controller. In *2024 5th International Conference on Intelligent Communication Technologies and Virtual Mobile Networks (ICICV)* (pp. 274–281). IEEE.

Lee, S., Jung, K., Koo, J., Lee, S., Choi, H., Jeon, J., Nam, J., & Choi, H. (2004, July 27). Braille display device using soft actuator. In *Smart structures and materials 2004: Electroactive polymer actuators and devices (EAPAD)* (Vol. 5385, pp. 368–379). SPIE.

Lewthwaite, S. (2014). Web accessibility standards and disability: Developing critical perspectives on accessibility. *Disability and Rehabilitation, 36*(16), 1375–1383.

Mamun, K. A., Nabid, R. A., Pranto, S. I., Lamim, S. M., Rahman, M. M., Mahammed, N., Huda, M. N., Sarker, F., & Khan, R. R. (2024). Smart reception: An artificial intelligence driven bangla language based receptionist system employing speech, speaker, and face recognition for automating reception services. *Engineering Applications of Artificial Intelligence, 136*, 108923.

Manzoor, S., Iftikhar, S., Ayub, I., Shahid, A., Haq, A. U., Muhammad, W., & Shafique, M. (2024). Range sensor-based assistive technology solutions for people with visual impairment: A review. *Disability and Rehabilitation: Assistive Technology, 19*(3), 576–584.

McCarthy, K. S., & Yan, E. F. (2024). Reading comprehension and constructive learning: Policy considerations in the age of artificial intelligence. *Policy Insights from the Behavioral and Brain Sciences, 11*(1), 19–26.

Michel-Villarreal, R., Vilalta-Perdomo, E., Salinas-Navarro, D. E., Thierry-Aguilera, R., & Gerardou, F. S. (2023). Challenges and opportunities of generative AI for higher education as explained by ChatGPT. *Education Sciences, 13*(9), 856.

Millett, P. (2021). Accuracy of speech-to-text captioning for students who are deaf or hard of hearing. *Journal of Educational, Pediatric & (Re) Habilitative Audiology, 25*.

Mineraud, J., Mazhelis, O., Su, X., & Tarkoma, S. (2016). A gap analysis of Internet-of-Things platforms. *Computer Communications, 89*, 5–16.

Nadarzynski, T., Knights, N., Husbands, D., Graham, C. A., Llewellyn, C. D., Buchanan, T., Montgomery, I., & Ridge, D. (2024). Achieving health equity through conversational AI: A roadmap for design and implementation of inclusive chatbots in healthcare. *PLOS Digital Health, 3*(5), e0000492.

Nasser, N., Ali, A. Y., Karim, L., & Al-Helali, A. (2024, April 9). Enhancing mobility for the visually impaired with AI and IoT-enabled mobile applications. ScienceOpen Preprints.

Nayak, S., & Das, R. K. (2020). Application of artificial intelligence (AI) in prosthetic and orthotic rehabilitation. In *Service robotics*. IntechOpen.

Ntoa, S., Margetis, G., Antona, M., & Stephanidis, C. (2022, October 1). Digital accessibility in intelligent environments. In *Human-automation interaction: Manufacturing, services and user experience* (pp. 453–475). Springer International Publishing.

Olawade, D. B., Bolarinwa, O. A., Adebisi, Y. A., & Shongwe, S. (2025). The role of artificial intelligence in enhancing healthcare for people with disabilities. *Social Science & Medicine, 364*, 117560.

Orynbay, L., Razakhova, B., Peer, P., Meden, B., & Emeršič, Ž. (2024). Recent advances in synthesis and interaction of speech, text, and vision. *Electronics, 13*(9), 1726.

Packin, N. G. (2021). Disability discrimination using AI systems, social media and digital platforms: Can we disable digital bias? *Social Media and Digital Platforms: Can We Disable Digital Bias, 8*(2).

Pancholi, S., Wachs, J. P., & Duerstock, B. S. (2024). Use of artificial intelligence techniques to assist individuals with physical disabilities. *Annual Review of Biomedical Engineering, 26*.

Pitt, K. M., & Ousley, C. L. (2024). Reimagining AAC designs for children during dynamic social situations by leveraging smart device design. *Augmentative and Alternative Communication, 20*, 1–7.

Premsai, I., & Thiyagu, T. M. (2024, March 13). IoT based wireless alert system for individuals with impaired hearing. In *2024 3rd International Conference on Sentiment Analysis and Deep Learning (ICSADL)* (pp. 662–666). IEEE.

Rodríguez-Fernández, A., Lobo-Prat, J., & Font-Llagunes, J. M. (2021). Systematic review on wearable lower-limb exoskeletons for gait training in neuromuscular impairments. *Journal of Neuroengineering and Rehabilitation, 18*(1), 22.

References

Sarker, I. H. (2021). Machine learning: Algorithms, real-world applications and research directions. *SN Computer Science, 2*(3), 160.

Satani, N., Patel, S., & Patel, S. (2020). AI powered glasses for visually impaired person. *International Journal of Recent Technology and Engineering (IJRTE), 9*(2), 416–421.

Selvi, A., Mounika, V., Rubika, V., & Uvadharanee, B. (2024, January 4). COLLEGEBOT: Virtual assistant system for enquiry using natural language processing. In *2024 2nd International Conference on Intelligent Data Communication Technologies and Internet of Things (IDCIoT)* (pp. 1407–1414). IEEE.

Sharma, V., Singh, V. M., & Thanneeru S. (2020, April 19). *Virtual assistant for visually impaired.* Available at SSRN 3580035.

Smaradottir, B. F., Håland, J. A., & Martinez, S. G. (2018). User evaluation of the smartphone screen reader VoiceOver with visually disabled participants. *Mobile Information Systems, 1*, 6941631.

Smith, P., & Smith, L. (2021). Artificial intelligence and disability: Too much promise, yet too little substance? *AI and Ethics, 1*(1), 81–86.

Soliman, M., Al-Shanfari, L. S., & Gulvady, S. (202). Sensory marketing and accessible tourism: An AI-generated article. *ROBONOMICS: The Journal of the Automated Economy, 4*, 53.

Sørensen, L., Johannesen, D. T., & Johnsen, H. M. (2024). Humanoid robots for assisting people with physical disabilities in activities of daily living: A scoping review. *Assistive Technology*, 1–7.

Spalteholz, L. (2012). *KeySurf-A keyboard web navigation system for persons with disabilities.* University of Victoria.

Sridhar, A., Poddar, R., Jain, M., & Kumar, P. (2023, August 25). Challenges faced by the employed Indian DHH community. In *IFIP Conference on Human-Computer Interaction* (pp. 201–223). Springer Nature Switzerland.

Srivastava, S., Varshney, A., Katyal, S., Kaur, R., & Gaur, V. (2021). A smart learning assistance tool for inclusive education. *Journal of Intelligent & Fuzzy Systems, 40*(6), 11981–11994.

Sumner, J., Lim, H. W., Chong, L. S., Bundele, A., Mukhopadhyay, A., & Kayambu, G. (2023). Artificial intelligence in physical rehabilitation: A systematic review. *Artificial Intelligence in Medicine*, 102693.

Tamdjidi, R. (2023). *ChatGPT as an assistive technology to enhance reading comprehension for individuals with ADHD.*

Tomlinson, B. J., Schuett, J. H., Shortridge, W., Chandran, J., & Walker, B. N. (2016, September 6). Talkin' about the weather: Incorporating TalkBack functionality and sonifications for accessible app design. In *Proceedings of the 18th International Conference on Human-Computer Interaction with Mobile Devices and Services* (pp. 377–386).

Tulshan, A. S., & Dhage, S. N. (2018, September 19–22). Survey on virtual assistant: Google assistant, Siri, Cortana, Alexa. In *Advances in Signal Processing and Intelligent Recognition Systems: 4th International Symposium SIRS 2018*, Bangalore, India. Revised Selected Papers 4 2019 (pp. 190–201). Springer Singapore.

van Balkom, L. J. (2022). *Elephant paths point the way to augmentative and alternative communication: Exploiting natural compensation in the brains and behaviour of people with multiple communicative disabilities.*

Venkatraman, S., Overmars, A., & Thong, M. (2021). Smart home automation—Use cases of a secure and integrated voice-control system. *Systems, 9*(4), 77.

Vinothkumar, J., & Karunamurthy, A. (2023). Recent advancements in artificial intelligence technology: Trends and implications. *Quing: International Journal of Multidisciplinary Scientific Research and Development, 2*(1), 1.

Vlahos, J. (2019). *Talk to me: Amazon, Google.* Random House.

Willingham, T. B., Stowell, J., Collier, G., & Backus, D. (2024). Leveraging emerging technologies to expand accessibility and improve precision in rehabilitation and exercise for people with disabilities. *International Journal of Environmental Research and Public Health, 21*(1), 79.

Yang, H. F., Ling, Y., Kopca, C., Ricord, S., & Wang, Y. (2022). Cooperative traffic signal assistance system for non-motorized users and disabilities empowered by computer vision and edge artificial intelligence. *Transportation Research Part C: Emerging Technologies, 145*, 103896.

Zhang, J., & Tao, D. (2020). Empowering things with intelligence: A survey of the progress, challenges, and opportunities in artificial intelligence of things. *IEEE Internet of Things Journal, 8*(10), 7789–7817.

Zhao, Y., Wu, S., Reynolds, L., & Azenkot, S. (2018). A face recognition application for people with visual impairments: Understanding use beyond the lab. In *Proceedings of the 2018 CHI Conference on Human Factors in Computing Systems* (pp. 1–14).

Chapter 4
AI-Driven Innovations in Assistive Technology for People with Disabilities

Abstract Artificial intelligence can transform assistive technologies for those with disabilities by improving accessibility, communication, and mobility. The amalgamation of AI and assistive technology has resulted in substantial progress, facilitating the creation of innovative solutions customized for various requirements. This chapter offers a comprehensive examination of AI-driven assistive technology, encompassing smart voice and speech recognition systems as well as AI-enhanced communication and learning tools. It examines sophisticated augmentative and alternative communication devices that improve interaction for those with speech disabilities. Moreover, AI-driven computer vision is essential for object recognition, assisting visually challenged individuals in traversing their environment. This chapter analyzes the influence of AI on prosthetic control, exoskeleton assistance, and intelligent wheelchairs, enhancing mobility and autonomy. Assistive technologies are continuously developing, thereby empowering individuals with disabilities and promoting a more inclusive and accessible world, by capitalizing on the capabilities of AI.

Keyword Assistive Technology · Communication · Speech recognition · Computer vision · Prosthesis · Exoskeletons

4.1 Introduction

The word physical disability denotes a category of disorders or diseases impacting the musculoskeletal or neural system, which hinders the control of physical objects and mobility in the environment. Assistive technology (AT) regularly empowers these groups to attain greater independence, engage in societal activities, and enhance self-sufficiency. Mobility devices including scooters, crutches, wheelchairs, orthotics, prosthetic limbs, and specialist home automation software are the most often utilized assistive technologies by people with physical disabilities (Korteling et al., 2021). For those with disabilities, the application of artificial intelligence (AI) could modify the benefits of assistive technology (AT). Artificial intelligence is a set of algorithms allowing machines to identify what people want, understand their surroundings, and react suitably to fulfill their goals (Sarker, 2021). A good life cannot be achieved without effective communication. For those with communication problems, this could be quite challenging. An assistive technology is a tool or equipment designed to enable individuals in daily tasks. Digital accessibility seeks to ensure that everyone including people with disabilities may access digital technologies and content. AT has greatly evolved in allowing people with disabilities more independence and a fulfilling life. Artificial intelligence (AI) is enabling these technologies to become ever more powerful and effective (Chemnad & Othman, 2024).

Prostheses employ artificial intelligence to assess user intents from physiological data and subsequently operate robotic actuators to complete actions such as opening and closing hands, moving fingers, and ramp and stair climbing. By measuring outside touch and sensory inputs, artificial intelligence helps prostheses send somatosensory signals to the brain. Prosthetic limbs equipped with biosensors like electromyograms (EMGs), force-sensitive resistors (FSRs), and mechanomyograms (MMGs) are being developed using artificial intelligence (Fernando et al., 2025). Like those gathered with electroencephalograms (EEGs) and electrocorticograms (ECoGs), brain-computer interface (BCI) technology analyzes human ideas from brain signals. This encoded intention then is used to run certain assistive devices (Zhao et al., 2018). People using lower limb prostheses combined with artificial intelligence can now more quickly adapt to different walking environments than those using non-intelligent prostheses (Ivanko et al., 2019).

Exoskeletons can be made more functional by artificial intelligence, which will help them to complete different locomotion tasks including climbing stairs and avoiding obstacles. Exoskeletons use artificial intelligence to interpret user stride and guide a robotic system to match. An exoskeleton can evaluate the necessary force when a person is unable to produce force or perform a given limb movement by using artificial intelligence alongside sensory information to increase power (Alarcon et al., 2024). Many research groups are looking at camera-equipped exoskeletons whereby artificial intelligence analyzes real-time images to identify movement and other traits to guide the best response to the surroundings (Kawas et al., 2016). AI-powered exoskeletons provide patients with a better perspective of their progress and increase their confidence, therefore improving rehabilitation.

While artificial intelligence analyzes this data to determine the best path forward, the sensors on a smart wheelchair let it sense and react to its surroundings. The intelligent wheelchair's intelligent features, brain-computer interface (BCI), voice recognition, and GPS navigation, increase users' freedom and safety. New artificial intelligence developments including computer vision, natural language processing, virtual reality, and augmented reality create innovative approaches for interacting with digital technology. These developments let individuals interact with technology utilizing picture classifying, brain activity detection, emotional understanding, and voice recognition. Using voice commands, such as lighting control, room temperature adjustment, stove operation, door opening, avatars, and chatbots, helps users connect with gadgets, therefore enabling the completion of ordinary everyday duties. For those with disabilities, voice assistants Alexa, Google Assistant, Cortana, and Siri help to improve communication. Just by talking through the microphone of their cell phones, they can acquire all the required information every day (Almufareh et al., 2024;Orynbay et al., 2024). This chapter will look at current developments in AI-driven assistive technologies for those with impairments. AI is creating a more inclusive digital environment, breaking down obstacles for people with disabilities, and changing accessibility.

4.2 Assistive Technologies

Assistive technologies are equipment or software meant to enable persons with impairments to complete tasks that could be challenging for them. Simple items like wheelchairs and hearing aids to more complex gadgets like prosthetic limbs and voice recognition software span these technologies (Pitt & Ousley, 2024). Assistive technologies seek to balance personal capacity with environmental needs. These technologies let persons with impairments increase their quality of life, increase their degree of freedom, and engage more actively in society (Packin, 2021). Visual technologies for those with visual impairments, color vision deficiency, or total blindness; auditory technologies for those with hearing disabilities; motor technologies for those exhibiting tremors, spasms, muscular bradykinesia, or impaired fine motor dexterity; and cognitive technologies for individuals facing challenges with reasoning, learning, memory, problem-solving, or attention. Diverse assistive technologies are available for individuals with disabilities. Disabled people rely heavily on assistive technology to boost their autonomy, movement, communication, and quality of life. People with disabilities can gain a lot from assistive technology. It can help them be more independent, communicate better, move around more freely, access information, find a job, participate in inclusive education and social activities, keep tabs on their health, personalize their experience, feel more empowered, and boost their self-esteem.

4.3 AI-Based Assistive Technologies

Artificial intelligence can be extensively utilized in all the assistive technologies for disabled individuals. The amalgamation of assistive technology with gadgets and machine learning within the domain of Artificial Intelligence of Things (AIoT) has undergone substantial progress. AI has changed the landscape of assistive technologies. New opportunities have arisen for those with impairments as a result of AI's capacity to learn, adapt, and make decisions. Smarter and more practical than older forms of assistive technology, devices driven by AI can evaluate data, identify trends, and provide predictions. The elimination of obstacles allows those with impairments to engage more fully in society. When used in this context, assistive technology (AT) can make daily tasks easier for people with disabilities (Fitria, 2022). Artificial intelligence can be incorporated into current assistive technologies, enhancing their intelligence and user-friendliness (Abdolrahmani et al., 2018; Smaradottir et al.,

2018; Tomlinson et al. 2016). A good example is the application of artificial intelligence (AI) in prosthetic limbs; these can then analyze the user's motions and make the necessary adjustments, making the overall experience more natural and comfortable. The next section explains about the various applications of AI-based assistive technology particularly for disabled individual.

4.3.1 Voice Recognition

AI and a variety of machine learning algorithms exhibit promising results in resolving issues related to speech identification, speech and speech recognition, and speech-to-text service applications, similar to a multitude of other scenarios that involve individuals with impairments. Most gadgets and technologies for assistive purposes combine machine learning with deep learning in innovative ways. Voice and sound generation technologies, as well as those that analyze written and spoken language, benefit greatly from it (Sharma et al., 2020). Artificial intelligence is essential for voice and speech recognition (Satani et al., 2020). Researchers discovered that deep learning techniques, especially BERT (Lee et al., 2004), can improve speech, voice, and speech recognition (Alkahtani, 2024). This field has seen the emergence of non-invasive brain-computer interfaces, which have led to much improved performance over traditional systems that process visual and auditory data (Selvi et al., 2024). They improve computer vision and NLP algorithms' categorization abilities by using novel deep learning approaches and structures. For children with childhood apraxia of speech (CAS), a speech-language pathologist is required for individualized treatment. Such sessions must occur over extended durations, placing significant demands on the time allocation of pathologists. Furthermore, numerous children requiring individualized sessions reside in rural regions, and the costs connected with therapy sessions hinder them from receiving the necessary support promptly (Sridhar et al., 2023).

Technology—more especially, artificial intelligence and machine learning—allows sufficient treatment for children with issues in their homes, therefore saving time and money. In a study by researcher (Premsai & Thiyagu, 2024), a solution was shown whereby a child's development was assessed by the therapist's assignment of speech exercises, which were subsequently examined using AI algorithms and fed back to the therapist. A comparable investigation reveals that the AI autonomously detects three categories of aberrant patterns linked to CAS: delays in sound production, erroneous phoneme pronunciation, and variable lexical stress (Ntoa et al., 2022). Particularly, challenges associated with quantifying inconsistent lexical stress are tackled through the utilization of deep neural network-based categorization techniques (Tulshan & Dhage, 2018). This tool aids in both diagnosis and therapy by employing the convolutional neural network (CNN) model to detect linguistic units that influence speech intelligibility (Mineraud et al., 2016) and voice recognition and production (Balgude et al., 2024). The latter study employed ways to obtain biosignals from muscle activation, brain activity, and articulatory activity to enhance accuracy.

Deep learning algorithms can be employed for individuals who stutter a speech impairment characterized by involuntary pauses or sound repetitions (Lewthwaite, 2014). The method employs a real-time program to capture an individual's voice, subsequently diagnoses and eliminates stammers by enhancing speech fluency, and ultimately generates a speech devoid of stuttering. A neural network model-generated amplitude threshold enhances the speech flow (Spalteholz, 2012).

4.3.2 Augmentative and Alternative Communication

Some individuals with disabilities might find it challenging to use speech as their main way of communicating, so they need to explore different methods or strategies to share their ideas. The objective of Augmented and Alternative Communication (AAC) is to optimize an individual's strengths to address their verbal communication deficiencies (Cave, 2024). The AAC system makes communication easier, improving overall quality of life. Different types of AAC are available, depending on the communication needs and capacities of the individual. Unassisted and aided ACC systems are the two main categories. There is no need for a tangible tool or aid while using an unassisted system, such as facial expressions or sign language. There are two main types of materials or technological instruments used by aided systems: (a) traditional methods of communication, such as picture boards, vocabulary cards, and communication books; and (b) modern methods, such as augmentative and alternative communication apps for smartphones, speech generators, and other communication aids.

The swift advancement of AI has recently created novel methods to tackle increasingly intricate issues, particularly in assisting individuals with complex communication requirements in surmounting obstacles (Millett, 2021). Powerful AI technologies can revolutionize augmentative and alternative communication (AAC) systems, including low-tech options utilizing words and symbols, as well as high-tech solutions that use computers to generate human voice output, particularly for education for disabled students (Balkom, 2022). To ensure that all students have equal access to high-quality education, image recognition technologies are indispensable. On an iPhone or iPad, the GoVisual software transforms images and videos into possibilities for reading and communication (Nayak & Das, 2020). This novel methodology integrates computer vision through image recognition technology (gathering images and videos), natural language processing tools for narrative development, and machine learning to facilitate object and shape identification for programming efficiency (Huq et al., 2024). Bringing together these three strategies encourages kids with disabilities to be independent and take charge of their learning in their educational institutions. AAC is a powerful tool for enhancing communication for those with significant speech challenges, including conditions like aphasia, articulation disorder, dysarthria, cluttering, apraxia of speech, and stuttering (Pancholi et al., 2024).

Movement impairments like multiple sclerosis, cerebral palsy, and Parkinson's disease, as well as cognitive problems like Down syndrome, dyslexia, and autism spectrum disorder (ASD) (Nadarzynski et al., 2024; Willingham et al., 2024), can also have an impact (Smith & Smith, 2021). One of the most notable AAC devices and technologies is assistive technology and devices that are designed to improve intelligibility (Bansal et al., 2024). Despite the present drawbacks of high-tech AAC, which are mostly related to inadequacies in recruitment, regulation, and infrastructure, their development is inevitable, and they will soon serve as a bridge between educators, assisted communicators, and their assistive technology. Communication is expected to change as a result of the integration of AAC devices with non-invasive brain-computer interface access techniques (Jaddoh et al., 2024). However, this shift will not be possible without strong neural imaging and machine learning technology.

4.3.3 *Speech Recognition and Natural Language Processing (NLP)*

Innovative technology has been created to transcribe spoken language into text. These programs immediately transcribe spoken conversation into text using sophisticated algorithms and AI. Speaking and writing provide an incredible means for anyone with disabilities or restrictions to express themselves and help everyone communicate easily. These devices create matching written text, analyze smartly using sophisticated voice recognition, and take in sound. This lets users interact with others, share ideas, and chat via writing. For those with speech and hearing difficulties, mobility disorders, dyslexia, and other conditions, speech-to-text tools are absolutely essential since they increase access and support inclusiveness. For persons with disabilities, Amberscript (Sørensen et al., 2024) is an amazing speech-to-text tool with various advantages. Equipped with modern technology and a simple interface, Amberscript offers a consistent and accurate way to translate spoken language into written text. Amberscript creates accurate transcriptions of spoken language by means of clever voice recognition and artificial intelligence technologies. It offers multiple integration choices so that customers may quickly include the tool in their chosen hardware or software. Google developed the smartphone software VoiceAccess (Rodríguez-Fernández et al., 2021). It can control a mobile phone with voice commands to send text, image, voice, and video messages. Windows includes default voice recognition programs for PCs. Apple now offers speech-assistive programs for device control via vocal commands. One can save time and effort by using Speechnotes, a trustworthy and secure web-based speech-to-text application, to transcribe audio and video recordings and dictate notes with ease (Olawade et al., 2025). With features like automatic capitalization, voice commands for punctuation and formatting, and easy import/export choices, Speechnotes provides a straightforward and gratifying experience for dictation and transcribing.

4.4 AI-Based Computer Vision for Object Recognition

AI-driven computer vision is transforming accessibility, allowing individuals with disabilities to engage more effortlessly with their environment. Object recognition technology uses machine learning to spot and categorize objects instantly, helping visually impaired users understand their surroundings through sound or touch feedback. AI-driven computer vision can recognize and articulate items inside the surroundings, and facilitates navigation for those with visual impairments by supplying information regarding their surrounding things (Kumar et al., 2024). These systems combine smart neural networks and edge computing to provide quick and precise detection, even in intricate or changing settings. Mobile apps, wearable tech, and smart glasses with these features boost navigation, help identify objects, and assist with tasks, fostering independence and safety. For example, Tobil is a specialized speech-generating gadget operated by ocular control for communication and Windows access (Willingham et al., 2024). Eye tracking is a technology that is employed to determine an individual's gaze on a computer screen. The computer might likewise be controlled using this technology. Users can direct it simply by glancing at it, rather than utilizing a standard mouse and keyboard.

Additionally, AI innovations allow for flexibility in meeting various user needs and identifying unique items or settings for enhanced usefulness. This innovative technology connects daily activities and promotes inclusivity, helping disabled individuals live more connected and independent lives. A new kind of wearable technology called "smart glasses" integrates AR and AI to give users an immersive, interactive, and hands-free experience (Yang et al., 2022). Users can effortlessly access information and engage with the digital environment with the help of these unique glasses, which include a display screen, camera, sensors, and smart algorithms. Using artificial intelligence algorithms, smart glasses can identify nearby objects and text. People who are visually impaired can now listen to descriptions of their surroundings, which greatly aids their navigation and offers them more independence. Smart glasses powered by AI can translate foreign languages in real time. Smart glasses with artificial intelligence can recognize faces, helping users identify people they encounter. This feature is especially helpful for those having trouble remembering or processing information since it allows them to learn more about the individuals they are interacting with, which improves their social connections.

4.5 AI-Enabled Prostheses Control

Recently, it has been estimated that more than one million amputations occur worldwide each year (Sumner et al., 2023). The predominant causes of amputation are significant trauma, muscular neoplasms, infection, and unregulated nerve tissue hypertrophy (Addy et al., 2023). Extensive research has been undertaken in recent decades to aid amputees through technology; nevertheless, artificial intelligence has markedly enhanced the realism of prosthetic devices, resembling human limbs. Artificial intelligence is focused on data and can be improved by collecting physiological information through biosensors such as EMG (Tamdjidi, 2023), EEG (McCarthy & Yan, 2024), and EOG (Botchu et al., 2024), as well as physical signals such as IMUs (McCarthy & Yan, 2024), MMG (Johnson et al., 2023), and FMG (Bozkurt et al., 2023). A significant decrease in categorization error was demonstrated in a study that used physiological data from both lower limbs that had been amputated and those that had not to forecast user intent (Chen & Zhu, 2023). The results of the experiment showed that including and attaching EMG sensors to the amputated limb, inertial measurement unit (IMU) sensors to the non-amputated leg, and an LDA classifier aids in controlling the lower limb prosthesis. Technology that allows for disarticulation of the shoulder joint and amputations above the wrist was developed by the Applied Physics Laboratory at Johns Hopkins University. Consequently, amputees can control certain prosthetic fingers, allowing them to perform manual functions. The researchers showed that to develop technology that would allow tetraplegic people to control two advanced prosthetic limbs using only brain impulses. At this point, prosthetics that use AI, like the Ottobock bebionic hands and the Össur i-Limb Ultra, can only do a limited number of grip patterns (Michel-Villarreal et al., 2023). These prostheses use EMG signals from the flexor and extensor muscles, allowing the user to control one movement, like opening and closing. These gadgets exhibited durability but were deficient in intuitiveness, perhaps elevating cognitive strain (Venkatraman et al., 2021). BCI-based prosthetics have demonstrated efficacy in prosthesis control (Vlahos, 2019).

Brain-computer interfaces (BCIs) can be implemented by invasive techniques like electrocorticography (ECoG), brain implants, electroencephalography (EEG), and electrooculography (EOG) (Cobb et al., 2020; Nasser et al., 2024). Induced brain-computer interfaces (BCIs) use either the steady-state visual evoked potential (SSVEP), the P300 evoked potential, or a combination of the two, and they are a subset of non-invasive BCIs (Almufareh et al. 2024; Orynbay et al., 2024) . Users must endure powerful visual flashes generated by stimulators to use stimulus-induced brain-computer interfaces, which have utilized artificial intelligence approaches by capitalizing on inputs from the occipital lobe (Almufareh et al., 2024). In contrast, nonstimulus BCIs employ methods like motor imagery in which users imagine moving their limbs without physically doing so and event-related desynchronization and synchronization signals in electroencephalograms. For people with disarticulated shoulders, a traditional prosthetic control system based on the detection of an EMG signal is inappropriate (Brotosaputro et al., 2024). A novel strategy that utilizes brain-machine interfaces called targeted muscle reinnervation (TMR) has the potential to address this problem.

Transcutaneous nerve reattachment (TMR) transfers any residual nerves from a severed limb to the muscle groups that have lost their connection to the severed arm. During this transfer process, the target muscles lose their nerve connections so that the nerves that once served the arm before amputation can reconnect and take over. The rejoined muscles then enhance the signals received from the severed nerves. Contemporary advancements in neural engineering enable individuals to use a prosthetic limb as required and perceive their environment (Srivastava et al., 2021). A wide range of feature extraction approaches and AI/ML methodologies are utilized in the investigation of lower and upper limb prosthesis regulation. In contrast to physical signals like IMUs, MMG, and FSR, the sEMG signal is non-invasive and responds quickly; hence, it was the primary signal employed in the tests. Researchers are actively exploring new deep learning architectures and moving away from traditional feature extraction methods for controlling prosthetics.

4.6 AI-Enabled Exoskeletons

Daily, disabled individuals encounter scenarios when their physical limitations hinder them, such as carrying substantial weights, performing repetitive tasks for prolonged durations, or conveying heavy items across extensive distances. People with physical disabilities or the elderly might face challenges with daily activities like walking, getting up from a chair, and climbing stairs. Stroke, which causes weakness in certain parts of the body, is the third most common cause of physical impairment in many nations. Problems with movement on the one side affect about 80% of stroke survivors. Around one-third of survivors that experience early paralysis of the legs do not recover basic skills, and between twenty-five percent and a quarter of all survivors require assistance when walking. Sixty-five percent of individuals that have experienced a stroke are unable to execute activities of daily living with their damaged hands after six months (Boppana, 2022). Consequently, the majority of individuals develop a lifelong dependency on others. Researchers are creating exoskeletons and robotic devices to address these challenges (Habuza et al., 2021).

Exoskeletons can be used to help lift and maintain loads, stabilize the body, and support a person's weight (Soliman et al., 2023). Some exoskeletons boost human strength and accuracy as helpful tools, while rehabilitation robots support stroke patients in regaining their lost abilities (Mamun et al., 2024). Regardless of their use, these wearable robotic systems must be specifically tailored to the unique anatomical configurations of individual humans to replicate structure and kinematics. Enabling exoskeletons to actively learn from human experiences in order to work in tandem with the user is a major difficulty. Exoskeletons directly interface with the human body; therefore, they must function based on patient data and acquire the necessary motor skills to ensure the safety and effectiveness of the training (Borgström & Luengprakarn, 2023). Artificial intelligence techniques can greatly enhance the computational ability of robot-assisted rehabilitation by learning from user experiences and anticipating unforeseen circumstances. Natural movement patterns and human intentions could be deduced by exoskeletons equipped with artificial intelligence capabilities (Deriba et al., 2024). Intelligent methodologies can assimilate knowledge from previous control protocols and adjust to evolving circumstances (Manzoor et al., 2024). Exoskeletons can connect with patients using signals from the body like EEG, EOG, FSR, MMG, EMG, and ground response force. Data from these sensors was used to build a machine learning model, therefore producing an intelligent robotic helper. By detecting electrical signals in the body and supporting joint movement, Cyberdyne's hybrid assistive limb (HAL) exoskeleton aids persons with lower limb problems from spinal cord injuries and strokes. Many studies involving SCI patients were conducted to investigate the way VR technologies and BCI might be coupled with artificial intelligence approaches. These studies reveal that a BCI can effectively run a device meant for lower limb rehabilitation. Designed for personalized physical rehabilitation therapy, a virtual reality training system was developed. This study gathered physiological data from the patient using a 3D graphical interface, therefore enhancing the interest of their rehabilitation process. Based on past medical records, the patient can follow a customized rehabilitation plan.

Furthermore, researchers proposed a bidirectional triboelectric sensor-based upper limb exoskeleton that might convey robotic actions to humans. Combining visual data with sophisticated decision-making for organizing its movement patterns allowed a fresh approach to assist the robot in better perceiving its environment. An RGB-D camera records data about the environment and helps the robot recognize ground objects with characteristics that might influence its movement. Researchers developed a four-limb neuroprosthetic exoskeleton for people with tetraplegia. The patient regained the ability to walk and use both arms with the help of this neuroprosthetic, which instantaneously controls an exoskeleton by capturing, transmitting, and interpreting brain impulses.

4.7 AI-Enabled Wheelchairs

The integration of AI technologies, sensors, and processors has facilitated the advancement of smart wheelchairs, enhancing the operation of classic power wheelchairs that require some upper limb motor control (Fig. 4.1). Many power wheelchair users, however, do not possess that degree of motor functionality, necessitating other control methods. By incorporating sensors that allow them to detect and react to varied situations with minimal to no human operator intervention, AI-enabled wheelchairs aim to improve upon traditional powered wheelchairs. To control power wheelchairs, researchers have investigated several HCI solutions that combine AI with restricted user movement. These include facial muscle movement, head gesture recognition, eye-tracking systems, joystick or head-joystick interfaces, finger movement tracking, tongue motion, and the traditional touchpad interface. Individuals with sensory or cognitive problems may encounter difficulties in implementing ideas.

4.7 AI-Enabled Wheelchairs

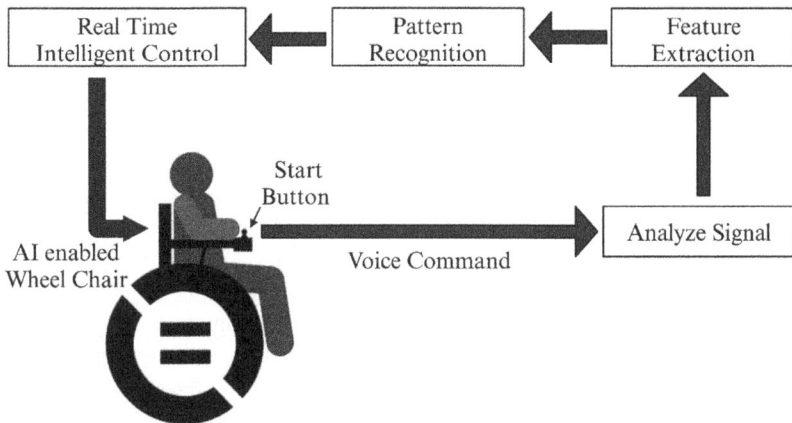

Fig. 4.1 AI-enabled voice instructions-based wheelchair navigation, enabling users to operate the wheelchair effectively

Voice instructions represent an attractive approach to wheelchair navigation, enabling users to operate the wheelchair effectively while remaining seated. Researchers demonstrated that a basic RGB camera paired with depth sensors can be used to control a wheelchair, verifying the location with three winks via AI software.

One study used a motorized wheelchair-mounted laptop with a 2D LIDAR sensor to feed data about the surrounding area into a SLAM (simultaneous localization and mapping) algorithm. It was autonomous vehicles that first used this technology. The SLAM instantaneously generated a map and inserted the wheelchair into it, enabling it to detect nearby barriers and things in motion and plot a course to its destination. Another study had the operator steer and throttle the wheelchair using a joystick. To train the neural network, the data collected from the three ultrasonic transducers mounted on the wheelchair was utilized. The neural network helped steer clear of obstacles and guided the way forward smoothly, avoiding any bumps along the journey. An innovative method was developed to assist motorized wheelchairs in following their users' daily routines and anticipating their destinations. The optimal prompting strategy was uncovered by a partially observable Markov decision process. This module evaluated users' skills in finding their way independently and chose the best sound cues to help them reach their destination. A unique collection of touch-based guidance algorithms was created to help wheelchairs move smoothly through busy environments. Power wheelchairs were created for people with paralysis from the neck down, and warmth or touch can activate the movement of the chairs. Users with paralysis-related speech problems could nonetheless communicate with the help of the smart wheelchairs' built-in visual perception and speech recognition software. A WT-SVM algorithm and a flexible hydrogel biosensor were used to construct a smart wheelchair prototype that responds to the user's eye movements.

4.8 Advanced Assistance by AI Through Human–Computer Interaction

Despite studies advocating for progress in HCI design, there remains potential for improvement in enhancing accessibility for individuals with physical limitations. Common electronic devices, such as televisions, laptops, tablets, and smartphones, can be challenging for this demographic to use with conventional input methods. Many efforts have been undertaken by the scientific community to address these difficulties. A study explored an HCI interface that examined photos of human faces and eyes to help people with upper limb movement disabilities use a keyboard, allowing them to choose the right key to press. A rapid-response control system has been created for spinal cord injury victims to manage their smart homes. A visual interface showcases several buttons, each connected to a unique command, that light up randomly from time to time. To communicate, the user needs to blink in time with an on-screen button. To identify the desired button and issue the command, the EOG signal is monitored for blinks (Fig. 4.2). Using skin-integrated electronics, researchers have developed a closed-loop human–machine interface system that can wirelessly record movements and provide haptic feedback using Wi-Fi and Bluetooth. Using this method could also lessen the need for expensive, cumbersome, and clumsy gadgets to provide feedback during rehabilitation exercises. Complete paralysis makes the use of a gesture recognition system impractical. To address this issue, a human–computer interaction system has been created that allows an individual to issue commands through breathing. These signals were collected by impulse radio ultrawideband sensors and subsequently fed into the machine learning system. Additionally, there is a promising future for assisting people with impairments through the translation of brain activity into control of assistive devices through the use of neural network brain-computer interfaces (NNBCI).

A gestural interface using machine vision was developed for people with upper extremity disabilities to help them with lab tasks that require handling components. A unique 3D particle filter framework was created using color and depth, showcasing its special descriptive features. This framework was woven into an interaction model that used spatial and motion data to tackle occlusions. The proposed method effectively addresses the issues of erroneous merging and inaccurate labeling commonly encountered during occlusion tracking. The identical feature-encoding method was employed to identify, monitor, and recognize users' hands. To understand ten common trackpad movements in a real-time pinch, stretch, swipe right, swipe left, scroll down, scroll up, pat, double click, single click, and OK, an innovative armband was created that uses electromyography (EMG) signals to detect hand gestures. To predict movements based on transitory electromyographic signals, a time-delayed artificial neural network is employed rather than conventional steady-state characteristics. The artificial neural network is executed on the microcontroller and requires under 0.2 ms to finalize. This method for operating computers or mobile devices can significantly assist people that have lost limbs.

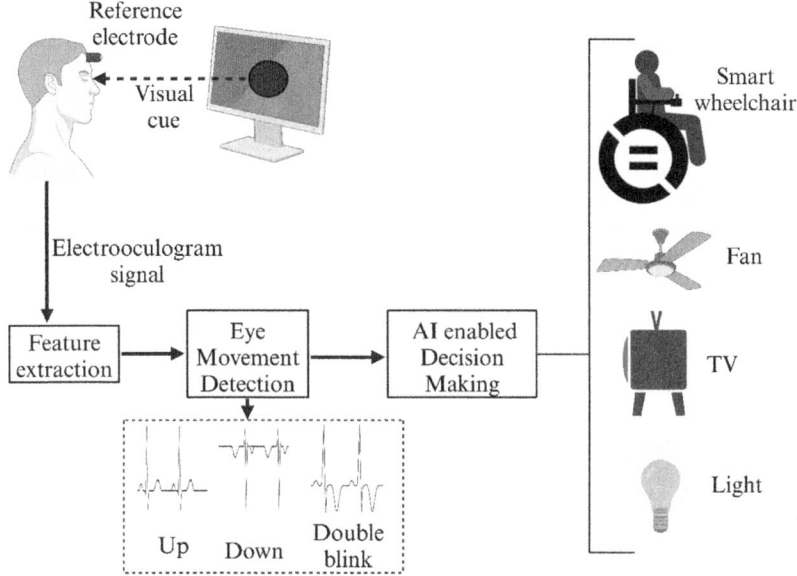

Fig. 4.2 AI-based smart electrooculogram-based system for home automation assisting disabled individuals

4.9 Conclusion

The advancement of AI-driven assistive devices represents a crucial progression toward a more accessible and inclusive future. These advances transcend mere convenience, significantly altering the lives of those with impairments. The amalgamation of AI and assistive technology has resulted in significant progress, improving communication, movement, and autonomy. AI-driven tools, including intelligent voice and speech recognition, sophisticated augmentative and alternative communication systems, and advanced learning assistive technologies, offer essential support. Furthermore, AI-enhanced computer vision facilitates object recognition for those with visual impairments, while AI-operated prosthetics, exoskeletons, and intelligent wheelchairs enhance mobility and independence. Utilizing AI's capabilities, assistive technologies are advancing, creating an environment where those with disabilities may navigate life more easily and confidently.

References

Abdolrahmani, A., Kuber, R., & Branham, S. M. (2018, October 8). "Siri Talks at You" an empirical investigation of voice-activated personal assistant (VAPA) usage by individuals who are blind. In *Proceedings of the 20th International ACM SIGACCESS Conference on Computers and Accessibility* (pp. 249–258).

Addy, T., Kang, T., Laquintano, T., & Dietrich, V. (2023). Who benefits and who is excluded?: Transformative learning, equity, and generative artificial intelligence. *Journal of Transformative Learning, 10*(2), 92–103.

Alarcon, R., Moreno, L., Martínez, P., & Macías, J. A. (2024). EASIER system. Evaluating a Spanish lexical simplification proposal with people with cognitive impairments. *International Journal of Human–Computer Interaction, 40*(5), 1195–1209.

Alkahtani, B. N. (2024). The impact of artificial intelligence on quality of life for deaf and hard of hearing students. *American Annals of the Deaf, 169*(4), 329–347.

Almufareh, M. F., Kausar, S., Humayun, M., & Tehsin, S. (2024). A conceptual model for inclusive technology: Advancing disability inclusion through artificial intelligence. *Journal of Disability Research, 3*(1), 20230060.

Balgude, S. D., Gite, S., Pradhan, B., & Lee, C. W. (2024). Artificial intelligence and machine learning approaches in cerebral palsy diagnosis, prognosis, and management: A comprehensive review. *PeerJ Computer Science, 10*, e2505.

Bansal, G., Chamola, V., Hussain, A., Guizani, M., & Niyato, D. (2024). Transforming conversations with AI—A comprehensive study of ChatGPT. *Cognitive Computation, 24*, 1–24.

Boppana, V. R. (2022). Impact of telemedicine platforms on patient care outcomes. *Innovative Engineering Sciences Journal, 2*(1).

Borgström, L., & Luengprakarn, T. (2023). Designing accessible medical information: Understanding the challenges and opportunities for blind and visually impaired individuals.

Botchu, B., Iyengar, K. P., & Botchu, R. (2024). Can ChatGPT empower people with dyslexia? *Disability and Rehabilitation: Assistive Technology, 19*(5), 2131–2132.

Bozkurt, A., Junhong, X., Lambert, S., Pazurek, A., Crompton, H., Koseoglu, S., Farrow, R., Bond, M., Nerantzi, C., Honeychurch, S., & Bali, M. (2023). Speculative futures on ChatGPT and generative artificial intelligence (AI): A collective reflection from the educational landscape. *Asian Journal of Distance Education, 18*(1), 53–130.

Brotosaputro, G., Supriyadi, A., & Jones, M. (2024). AI-powered assistive technologies for improved accessibility. *International Transactions on Artificial Intelligence, 3*(1), 76–84.

Cave, R. (2024). *How people living with motor neurone disease use personalised automatic speech recognition technology to support social interaction* (Doctoral dissertation, UCL (University College London)).

Chemnad, K., & Othman, A. (2024). Digital accessibility in the era of artificial intelligence—Bibliometric analysis and systematic review. *Frontiers in Artificial Intelligence, 7*, 1349668.

Chen, B., & Zhu, X. (2023). Integrating generative AI in knowledge building. *Computers and Education: Artificial Intelligence, 5*, 100184.

Cobb, C., Surbatovich, M., Kawakami, A., Sharif, M., Bauer, L., Das, A., & Jia, L. (2020). How risky are real users' {IFTTT} applets? In *Sixteenth Symposium on Usable Privacy and Security (SOUPS 2020)* (pp. 505–529).

Deriba, F. G., Wubineh, B. Z., & Teka, M. Z. (2024, November 18). Review of AI technologies for enhancing the lives of visually impaired individuals: Applications, outcomes, and future directions. In *2024 International Conference on Information and Communication Technology for Development for Africa (ICT4DA)* (pp. 241–246). IEEE.

Fernando, S., Ndukwe, C., Virdee, B., & Djemai, R. (2025). Image recognition tools for blind and visually impaired users: An emphasis on the design considerations. *ACM Transactions on Accessible Computing, 18*(1), 1–21.

Fitria, T. N. (2022). Utilizing text-to-speech technology: Natural reader in teaching pronunciation. *JETLEE: Journal of English Language Teaching, Linguistics, and Literature, 2*(2), 70–78.

Habuza, T., Navaz, A. N., Hashim, F., Alnajjar, F., Zaki, N., Serhani, M. A., & Statsenko, Y. (2021). AI applications in robotics, diagnostic image analysis and precision medicine: Current limitations, future trends, guidelines on CAD systems for medicine. *Informatics in Medicine Unlocked, 1*(24), 100596.

References

Huq, S. M., Maskeliūnas, R., & Damaševičius, R. (2024). Dialogue agents for artificial intelligence-based conversational systems for cognitively disabled: A systematic review. *Disability and Rehabilitation: Assistive Technology, 19*(3), 1059–1078.

Ivanko, D., Ryumin, D., & Karpov, A. (2019). Automatic lip-reading of hearing impaired people. *The International Archives of the Photogrammetry, Remote Sensing and Spatial Information Sciences, 42*, 97–101.

Jaddoh, A., Loizides, F., Rana, O., & Syed, Y. A. (2024). Interacting with smart virtual assistants for individuals with dysarthria: A comparative study on usability and user preferences. *Applied Sciences, 14*(4), 1409.

Johnson, C., Smart, K., & Mahar, P. (2023). Is there a place for generative artificial intelligence in special education? *National Social Science Technology Journal, 48*.

Kawas, S., Karalis, G., Wen, T., & Ladner, R. E. (2016, October 23). Improving real-time captioning experiences for deaf and hard of hearing students. In *Proceedings of the 18th International ACM SIGACCESS Conference on Computers and Accessibility* (pp. 15–23).

Korteling, J. H., van de Boer-Visschedijk, G. C., Blankendaal, R. A., Boonekamp, R. C., & Eikelboom, A. R. (2021). Human-versus artificial intelligence. *Frontiers in Artificial Intelligence, 4*, 622364.

Kumar, A., Singh, M., Singh, M., Ramprabu, J., Dubey, A., & Mujoo, S. (2024, March 11). A novel electronic wheel chair design using artificial intelligence assisted smart sensors and controller. In *2024 5th International Conference on Intelligent Communication Technologies and Virtual Mobile Networks (ICICV)* (pp. 274–281). IEEE.

Lee, S., Jung, K., Koo, J., Lee, S., Choi, H., Jeon, J., Nam, J., & Choi, H. (2004, July 27). Braille display device using soft actuator. In *Smart structures and materials 2004: Electroactive polymer actuators and devices (EAPAD)* (Vol. 5385, pp. 368–379). SPIE.

Lewthwaite, S. (2014). Web accessibility standards and disability: Developing critical perspectives on accessibility. *Disability and Rehabilitation, 36*(16), 1375–1383.

Mamun, K. A., Nabid, R. A., Pranto, S. I., Lamim, S. M., Rahman, M. M., Mahammed, N., Huda, M. N., Sarker, F., & Khan, R. R. (2024). Smart reception: An artificial intelligence driven bangla language based receptionist system employing speech, speaker, and face recognition for automating reception services. *Engineering Applications of Artificial Intelligence, 136*, 108923.

Manzoor, S., Iftikhar, S., Ayub, I., Shahid, A., Haq, A. U., Muhammad, W., & Shafique, M. (2024). Range sensor-based assistive technology solutions for people with visual impairment: A review. *Disability and Rehabilitation: Assistive Technology, 19*(3), 576–584.

McCarthy, K. S., & Yan, E. F. (2024). Reading comprehension and constructive learning: Policy considerations in the age of artificial intelligence. *Policy Insights from the Behavioral and Brain Sciences, 11*(1), 19–26.

Michel-Villarreal, R., Vilalta-Perdomo, E., Salinas-Navarro, D. E., Thierry-Aguilera, R., & Gerardou, F. S. (2023). Challenges and opportunities of generative AI for higher education as explained by ChatGPT. *Education Sciences, 13*(9), 856.

Millett, P. (2021, January 1). Accuracy of speech-to-text captioning for students who are deaf or hard of hearing. *Journal of Educational, Pediatric & (Re) Habilitative Audiology, 25*.

Mineraud, J., Mazhelis, O., Su, X., & Tarkoma, S. (2016). A gap analysis of Internet-of-Things platforms. *Computer Communications, 89*, 5–16.

Nadarzynski, T., Knights, N., Husbands, D., Graham, C. A., Llewellyn, C. D., Buchanan, T., Montgomery, I., & Ridge, D. (2024). Achieving health equity through conversational AI: A roadmap for design and implementation of inclusive chatbots in healthcare. *PLOS Digital Health, 3*(5), e0000492.

Nasser, N., Ali, A. Y., Karim, L., & Al-Helali, A. (2024, April 9). Enhancing mobility for the visually impaired with AI and IoT-enabled mobile applications. ScienceOpen Preprints.

Nayak, S., & Das, R. K. (2020, October 7). Application of artificial intelligence (AI) in prosthetic and orthotic rehabilitation. In *Service robotics*. IntechOpen.

Ntoa, S., Margetis, G., Antona, M., & Stephanidis, C. (2022, October 1). Digital accessibility in intelligent environments. In *Human-automation interaction: Manufacturing, services and user experience* (pp. 453–475). Springer International Publishing.

Olawade, D. B., Bolarinwa, O. A., Adebisi, Y. A., & Shongwe, S. (2025). The role of artificial intelligence in enhancing healthcare for people with disabilities. *Social Science & Medicine, 1*(364), 117560.

Orynbay, L., Razakhova, B., Peer, P., Meden, B., & Emeršič, Ž. (2024). Recent advances in synthesis and interaction of speech, text, and vision. *Electronics, 13*(9), 1726.

Packin, N. G. (2021). Disability discrimination using AI systems, social media and digital platforms: Can we disable digital bias? *Social Media and Digital Platforms: Can We Disable Digital Bias, 8*(2).

Pancholi, S., Wachs, J. P., & Duerstock, B. S. (2024). Use of artificial intelligence techniques to assist individuals with physical disabilities. *Annual Review of Biomedical Engineering, 26*.

Pitt, K. M., & Ousley, C. L. (2024). Reimagining AAC designs for children during dynamic social situations by leveraging smart device design. *Augmentative and Alternative Communication*, 1–7.

Premsai, I., & Thiyagu, T. M. (2024, March 13) IoT based wireless alert system for individuals with impaired hearing. In *2024 3rd International Conference on Sentiment Analysis and Deep Learning (ICSADL)* (pp. 662–666). IEEE.

Rodríguez-Fernández, A., Lobo-Prat, J., & Font-Llagunes, J. M. (2021). Systematic review on wearable lower-limb exoskeletons for gait training in neuromuscular impairments. *Journal of Neuroengineering and Rehabilitation, 18*(1), 22.

Sarker, I. H. (2021). Machine learning: Algorithms, real-world applications and research directions. *SN Computer Science, 2*(3), 160.

Satani, N., Patel, S., & Patel, S. (2020). AI powered glasses for visually impaired person. *International Journal of Recent Technology and Engineering (IJRTE), 9*(2), 416–421.

Selvi, A., Mounika, V., Rubika, V., & Uvadharanee, B. (2024, January 4). COLLEGEBOT: Virtual assistant system for enquiry using natural language processing. In *2024 2nd International Conference on Intelligent Data Communication Technologies and Internet of Things (IDCIoT)* (pp. 1407–1414). IEEE.

Sharma, V., Singh, V. M., & Thanneeru, S. (2020). Virtual assistant for visually impaired. Available at SSRN 3580035.

Smaradottir, B. F., Håland, J. A., & Martinez, S. G. (2018). User evaluation of the smartphone screen reader VoiceOver with visually disabled participants. *Mobile Information Systems, 2018*(1), 6941631.

Smith, P., & Smith, L. (2021). Artificial intelligence and disability: Too much promise, yet too little substance? *AI and Ethics, 1*(1), 81–86.

Soliman, M., Al-Shanfari, L. S., & Gulvady, S. (2023). Sensory marketing and accessible tourism: An AI-generated article. *ROBONOMICS: The Journal of the Automated Economy, 4*, 53.

Sørensen, L., Johannesen, D. T., & Johnsen, H. M. (2024). Humanoid robots for assisting people with physical disabilities in activities of daily living: A scoping review. *Assistive Technology, 5*, 1–7.

Spalteholz, L. (2012). KeySurf-A keyboard Web navigation system for persons with disabilities. University of Victoria (Canada).

Sridhar, A., Poddar, R., Jain, M., & Kumar, P. (2023, August 25). Challenges faced by the employed Indian DHH community. In *IFIP Conference on Human-Computer Interaction* (pp. 201–223). Springer Nature Switzerland.

Srivastava, S., Varshney, A., Katyal, S., Kaur, R., & Gaur, V. (2021). A smart learning assistance tool for inclusive education. *Journal of Intelligent & Fuzzy Systems, 40*(6), 11981–11994.

Sumner, J., Lim, H. W., Chong, L. S., Bundele, A., Mukhopadhyay, A., & Kayambu, G. (2023). Artificial intelligence in physical rehabilitation: A systematic review. *Artificial Intelligence in Medicine, 2*, 102693.

References

Tamdjidi, R. (2023). ChatGPT as an assistive technology to enhance reading comprehension for individuals with ADHD.

Tomlinson, B. J., Schuett, J. H., Shortridge, W., Chandran, J., & Walker, B. N. (2016, September 6). Talkin' about the weather: Incorporating TalkBack functionality and sonifications for accessible app design. In *Proceedings of the 18th International Conference on Human-Computer Interaction with Mobile Devices and Services* (pp. 377–386).

Tulshan, A. S., & Dhage, S. N. (2018, September 19–22). Survey on virtual assistant: Google assistant, siri, cortana, alexa. In *Advances in Signal Processing and Intelligent Recognition Systems: 4th International Symposium SIRS 2018, Bangalore, India.* Revised Selected Papers 4 2019 (pp. 190–201). Springer Singapore.

van Balkom, L. J. (2022). Elephant paths point the way to augmentative and alternative communication: Exploiting natural compensation in the brains and behaviour of people with multiple communicative disabilities.

Venkatraman, S., Overmars, A., & Thong, M. (2021). Smart home automation—use cases of a secure and integrated voice-control system. *Systems, 9*(4), 77.

Vlahos, J. (2019). *Talk to me: Amazon, Google*. Random House.

Willingham, T. B., Stowell, J., Collier, G., & Backus, D. (2024). Leveraging emerging technologies to expand accessibility and improve precision in rehabilitation and exercise for people with disabilities. *International Journal of Environmental Research and Public Health, 21*(1), 79.

Yang, H. F., Ling, Y., Kopca, C., Ricord, S., & Wang, Y. (2022). Cooperative traffic signal assistance system for non-motorized users and disabilities empowered by computer vision and edge artificial intelligence. *Transportation Research Part c: Emerging Technologies, 1*(145), 103896.

Zhao, Y., Wu, S., Reynolds, L., & Azenkot, S. (2018, April 21). A face recognition application for people with visual impairments: Understanding use beyond the lab. In *Proceedings of the 2018 CHI Conference on Human Factors in Computing Systems* (pp. 1–14).

Chapter 5
Personalized Support for People with Disabilities Through Generative AI

Abstract As artificial intelligence (AI) progressively transforms disability support, its importance in personalized assistive technology is growing markedly. AI-driven personalized support solutions mitigate the obstacles encountered by those with impairments, facilitating enhanced access to education, healthcare, and social engagement. The amalgamation of AI with personalized assistive technology has resulted in significant improvements, offering customized help that improves autonomy and quality of life. Innovations including virtual assistant chatbots, wearable gadgets, predictive analytics, and automated systems are revolutionizing disability support, enhancing its interactivity and responsiveness. This chapter examines the integration of AI-driven personalized assistive technologies, emphasizing significant applications including AI-enabled motion detection for improved accessibility and visual analysis for tailored support. Furthermore, it explores AI-driven personalized healthcare solutions, encompassing virtual assistant chatbots for patient assistance and education, telemonitoring via wearable devices, predictive disease analytics for customized therapy, and automated appointment scheduling. These developments not only improve accessibility but also establish a more cohesive and responsive support structure for those with impairments. Through the utilization of AI's capabilities, assistive technology is advancing, promoting a more inclusive society in which those with disabilities may navigate life with enhanced ease and autonomy.

Keyword Personalised support · IoT · Motion detection · Visual analysis · Chatbot · Telepatient

5.1 Introduction

According to the World Health Organization, approximately 15% of the global population, equating to almost 190 million individuals, is believed to have a kind of disability. The WHO suggests that this figure is expected to rise, especially due to the increasing prevalence of chronic health conditions and the global aging population.

Disabilities, whether temporary or permanent, encompass a wide range of distinct demands, constraints, and health issues. Additionally, the likelihood of encountering certain disability may increase with aging (World Health Organization, 2011). The United Nations Convention on the Rights of Persons with Disabilities (CRPD) defines disability not as an inherent trait of an individual, but as a consequence of environmental impediments and societal practices that affect individuals with disabilities. This interaction lets individuals to avoid totally and equitably engaging as citizens. Therefore, tackling the difficulties experienced by people with disabilities improves their general social interaction. For people with disabilities, assistive technology (AT) enables fast solutions for problems in their daily lives. Supporting their learning and participation in the economy and society with respect, assistive technology helps people live on their own, stay healthy, and be productive (King & Martínez, 2020).

Assistive technology is a spectrum of services, tools, approaches, tactics, and procedures meant to enable people to overcome obstacles and restrictions resulting from impairments or incapacities. It emphasizes for those with disabilities the value of freedom, better living conditions, and community connection. Examples of assistive technology include customized hearing aids, memory aids, spectacles, wheelchairs, pill organizers, and communication devices. Assistive technology has made substantial advancements through the integration of AI, IoT devices, and machine learning. Employing AI methodologies, especially machine learning, to analyze the vast amounts of data generated by IoT devices facilitates the extraction of insights and simplifies decision-making (Sung et al., 2021).

When implemented in assistive technology, AI with IoT facilitates the development of various personalized innovative solutions to tackle disability challenges. Some solutions in this area are navigation systems designed for the visually impaired, voice assistants tailored for individuals with disabilities (Polyakov et al., 2018), remote health monitoring tools (Qian et al., 2021), telemedicine and telehealth services (Carter et al., 2021), communication systems that incorporate sign language, memory aids for cognitive impairments (Jacob et al., 2021), and a range of smart devices like medication dispensers and wheelchairs (Soma et al., 2018). Mary Pat Radabaugh, the former director of IBM's National Support Center for Individuals with Disabilities in 1988, remarked that technology provides significant advantages for those in need: "For individuals without disabilities, technology simplifies life." Technology enables those with disabilities to lead functional lives (Bryant & Seok, 2017).

5.2 AI in Assistive Technology

The World Health Organization defines assistive technology as a comprehensive phase that includes any system or service associated with assistive products and services, with the goal of reducing or removing constraints and limits faced by individuals owing to disabilities or incapacities. According to the Assistive Technology Industry Association, any device created to assist those with impairments is classified

5.2 AI in Assistive Technology

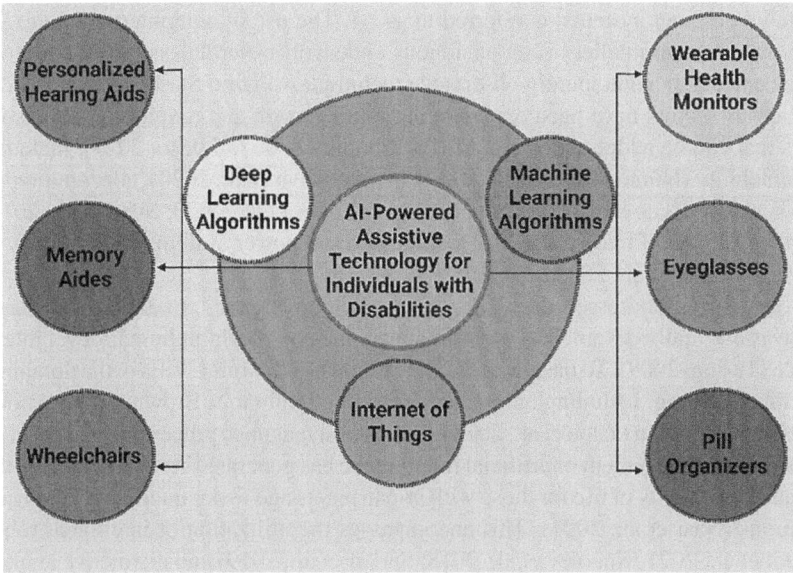

Fig. 5.1 Assistive technologies for individuals with disabilities integrating deep learning, machine learning, and IoT with disabilities

as assistive technology. This encompasses both tangible and digital resources. These offerings come from blending AT and AIoT (AI with IoT) (Zhang & Tao, 2020). Industry 4.0 acts as a partner in boosting AT. The rise of personalized devices powered by AI and the IoT will improve the quality of life for many people who depend on assistive technologies (Fig. 5.1). Conversely, individuals with impairments can gain access to all the services inside the Industry 4.0 framework through the utilization of personalized assistive technologies (Viel et al., 2018). The design and functionality of personalized assistive technologies, aimed at enhancing the overall participation of individuals with impairments, are critically significant.

The Artificial Intelligence of Things comes from blending the IoT with AI methods (Sopelsa Neto et al., 2021). The phrase IoT denotes a network of interconnected computing devices, networks, and sensors capable of continuously collecting valuable data (Leithardt et al., 2020). Analyzing the collected data using AI models, especially via ML, underscores its importance. Certain instances necessitate the application of DL to examine the gathered data for the extraction of pertinent information to inform decision-making (Frizzo Stefenon et al., 2020; Kasburg & Stefenon, 2019; Dingli & Fournier, 2017). The implementation of machine learning techniques demonstrates the potential for providing personalized assistance to disabled individuals by enhancing efficiency (Salazar et al., 2021; Salazar et al., 2020). In 1956, at the inaugural AI conference at Dartmouth College, the term was first used by John McCarthy, usually regarded as the progenitor of artificial intelligence (Dick, 2024). According to McCarthy, the study and development of intelligent devices, namely computer systems, is referred to as AI. The use of computers in the examination of human intellect is an analogous endeavor; nevertheless, artificial intelligence extends beyond merely observable techniques (Frizzo Stefenon et al., 2020). Numerous sectors have been experiencing rapid growth and require dynamic solutions that can be addressed using AI (Paz Santana & de la Iglesia 2021), including sustainability (Ninno Muniz et al., 2020), health (Silva et al., 2020), telecommunication systems (Kaur et al., 2021), data privacy (Lopes et al., 2020; Silva et al., 2019), electric vehicles (Pinto et al., 2021), and electrical power systems (Stefenon et al., 2021; Stefenon et al., 2022a, 2022b).

Alan Turing addressed the issue, "Can machines think?", in 1950. The Turing test was originally designed to assess if a machine could exhibit human-level intelligence (Turing, 2009). To pass this test, the system must exhibit skills in the domain of machine learning, including automated reasoning (Kumar & Brown, 2018), knowledge representation (Zhou et al., 2018), and natural language processing (Tissot et al., 2020). The advancement of artificial intelligence has generated several resources that enhance the quality of life for those with impairments and foster intelligent healthcare solutions (Nasr et al., 2021). This encompasses the utilization of intelligent robots (Fuadi et al., 2021; Kearney et al., 2018; Sarkar et al., 2019) and distinctive applications for sign language (Caliwag et al., 2018). In the domain of artificial intelligence, machine learning seeks to create models and software that can autonomously learn from data (Zikky et al., 2017). These programs must possess the capability to learn from their errors and independently evolve, devoid of human interference. These models are utilized in the Internet of Things (IoT) sector for processing and analyzing huge data volumes collected by devices, facilitating automatic pattern detection and extracting valuable insights from this data. Humans would struggle to do such a task manually. Adaptive neuro-fuzzy inference system (ANFIS) (Frizzo Stefenon et al., 2019), group method of data handling (GMDH) (Stefenon et al., 2022), convolutional neural networks (CNNs) (Stefenon et al., 2021), ensemble learning methods (Corso et al., 2021), k-nearest neighbors (K-NN) (Stefenon et al., 2020), long short-term memory (LSTM) (Fernandes et al., 2022), and echo state networks (Vieira et al., 2022) include machine learning models (Frizzo Stefenon et al., 2020).

Deep learning is a subfield of machine learning. The discipline focused on the examination of deep neural networks is termed deep learning. Deep learning, while employing multilayer neural networks for analysis and computation, is fundamentally data driven, akin to machine learning (Chang, 2015). Deep architectures surpass shallow structures in heuristic assessments and experimental results in contemporary applications addressing complex issues such as vision, natural language understanding, and large-scale data processing (Kim & Gofman, 2018). These models can be used for prediction (Salazar et al., 2020), classification (Stefenon et al., 2022), and optimization tasks (Frizzo Stefenon et al., 2020).

5.3 Application of AI for Personalized Support to Disabled

5.3.1 Motion Detection for Enhanced Accessibility

AI-enabled computer vision algorithms can recognize and monitor users' motions, allowing assistive equipment to adapt lighting, temperature, and other environmental variables to suit individual needs and preferences (Fig. 5.2). This technology improves tailored support for individuals with disabilities in significant manners (Sharma et al., 2024). Motion detection systems powered by AI work really well for spotting falls, especially for people having difficulty moving, like older adults or those living with Parkinson's disease. These devices can rapidly detect abrupt changes in mobility, therefore alerting emergency responders or caregivers for fast assistance (Silva de Lima et al., 2017). For those with impairments, including the elderly and those living with dementia, they are crucial in organizing their activities. Examining movement patterns helps these systems reveal activity levels and behaviors, therefore enabling caretakers or family members to provide the appropriate assistance (Mora et al., 2019).

Artificial intelligence-powered motion detection systems can identify and track objects throughout designated areas while recognizing wheelchairs and mobility aids among them. Through this capability, the device aids navigation for people with disabilities to improve their engagement with environmental elements (Sahoo & Choudhury, 2023). Assistive devices learn to detect and respond to specified hand

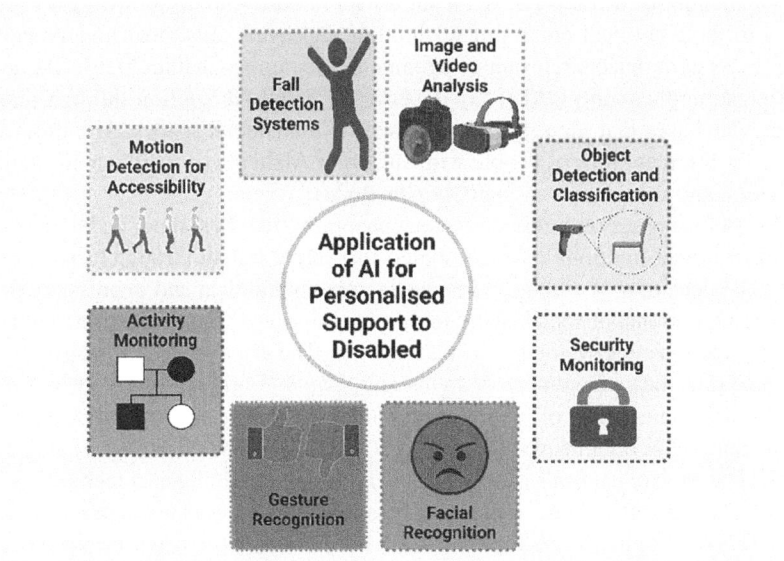

Fig. 5.2 Various applications of personalized support of AI for people with disabilities

signals and head gestures through the advanced artificial intelligence method of gesture recognition (Hashi et al., 2018). Users enjoy better device and environment interaction through these advancements which boosts their autonomy. Artificial intelligence (AI) systems which detect motion analyze all movements of objects and human beings to keep watch over homes and businesses (Al-Dulaimi, 2021). These security systems provide quick response for notifying customers about possible security hazards or criminal activity. People having disabilities find great value in AI technology which can observe and track motion-based activities in selected situations. These technological systems give vital information to users while providing assistance and better navigation which together increase the overall quality of life during everyday activities. New AI advancements showcase the way personal assistance tools receive transfiguration through AI-based developments (Fig. 5.2).

5.3.2 Visual Analysis for Accessibility

Computer vision algorithms created using artificial intelligence technology analyze pictures and videos obtained by cameras to give meaningful assessments about their content (Fig. 5.2) (Badidi et al., 2023). Following a kitchen picture analysis, an AI system can provide vocal instructions about preparing the designated dish. This technology delivers multiple groundbreaking applications to boost accessibility options for users with disabilities. AI technology performs visual analysis which leads to the identification of things within a particular environment consisting of furniture appliances and equipment (Ficocelli & Nejat, 2012). People with disabilities gain better access to their physical environment through improved situational understanding since the system detects relevant environmental features (Challa, 2023). The most widespread application of AI today depends on facial recognition through photographic databases that identify people based on their facial shapes. The improved face recognition abilities of people with autism or Alzheimer's lead to better family interaction and caregiver bonding (Chopde, 2024).

AI systems possess emotion detection capabilities that help them understand and recognize human emotions and face-related non-verbal signals through facial expressions. The detection of emotions enables people with autism and depression along with other emotional or social issues to develop improved communication and interpersonal relationships (Marechal et al. 2019 Mar). The visual composition of a scene, encompassing the arrangement of items and spatial configurations, can be evaluated through the analysis of pictures and videos. For those with visual disabilities, these technologies offer insightful analysis of spatial layouts that facilitate navigating greatly. Descriptive captions or text created by artificial intelligence technology for visual content enables those with visual disabilities to access knowledge in unique ways. This quality helps one to understand and interact with visual material (Saini et al., 2024). One adaptable tool that helps persons with impairments in several ways is artificial intelligence-powered image and video analysis. These technologies improve independence and quality of life using customized assistance in navigation, communication, and engagement using visual information from images and videos.

5.4 Personalized Healthcare Solutions

5.4.1 AI Chatbots for Patient Support and Education

Particularly for those with disabilities, chatbots can act as virtual assistants customizing medical aid and education to fit every person's preference and needs. By use of machine learning and natural language processing (NLP), chatbots can learn from patient interactions and adapt their responses to reflect the language and style of handicapped individuals, hence generating a more natural and interesting user experience (Aggarwal et al., 2023; Kurniawan et al., 2024). Virtual assistant chatbots provide 24/7 tailored help that would be quite beneficial for patients who cannot access their healthcare providers during regular office hours. Chatbots are always available; hence, patients may get the required assistance anytime they need it. Moreover, using medical record analysis and risk factor analysis, chatbots acting as virtual assistants can customize health recommendations and information for each unique individual (Abd Rahman et al., 2020). Reviewing a patient's medical history helps one decide on the appropriate course of treatment and preventative measures for a handicap (Calvaresi et al., 2023). By offering customized reminders and medical advice, chatbots—as virtual assistants—can let persons with disabilities understand and follow their treatment plans (Bertagnolli et al., 2020). Based on their food choices and activity level, a chatbot can offer healthy diet programs and exercise regimens to patients with disabilities. From minor ailments to long-term problems and mental health concerns, machine learning and artificial intelligence drive a rainbow of online chatbots offering tailored health information and support (Chen and Decary 2020; Magalhaes Azevedo & Kieffer, 2021; You et al., 2023).

5.4.2 Real-Time and Telepatient Monitoring with Wearables

Wearable devices and sensors enable real-time patient monitoring and remote care, helping healthcare professionals keep an eye on vital signs and biometric data, especially for individuals with disabilities (He & Lee, 2021). Smartwatches can monitor a patient's heart rate and blood pressure, sending this information wirelessly to a central monitoring station for analysis and interpretation by healthcare specialists. Wearable sensors, which are compact and portable, can monitor the vital signs and health metrics of individuals with disabilities, including heart rate, blood pressure, respiration rate, blood oxygen saturation, body temperature, and physical activity.

The data can be wirelessly transferred to a central monitoring station for comprehensive examination (Nguyen et al., 2023). Moreover, the vital signs of disabled patients can be monitored in real time with programs that leverage smartphone sensors and wearable technology. They can monitor dietary intake, sleep patterns, and exercise regimens, and they can also offer guidance on enhancing health management (Hrabovska et al., 2023). Additionally, the vital signs of handicapped patients can be monitored in real time using smart home devices such as speakers and thermostats. From the employment of wearable gadgets and sensors for real-time patient monitoring (Wang et al., 2023), patients and healthcare professionals both can gain much especially for people with disabilities. Patients will feel more protected and comfortable knowing their health is under constant observation and that any changes in their condition will be noted right away. By tracking the evolution of their diseases and better knowing their health needs, medical professionals enable more individualized and careful treatment (Mukkamala et al., 2021). Moreover, wearable sensors and technologies for real-time patient monitoring can streamline some procedures, therefore lessening the burden on medical practitioners and the possibility of mistakes (Zamani et al., 2023).

5.4.3 *Personalized Treatment Recommendations*

Two main objectives of healthcare data-driven tailored treatment recommendations which are especially important for people with disabilities are improved patient outcomes and lower medical costs. Deep learning algorithms can be used to evaluate a patient's genomic, genetic, demographic, and lifestyle data among other forms of patient data to forecast their reaction to different therapies. Whole-genome sequencing, gene expression patterns, and single-nucleotide polymorphisms (SNPs) (Liu et al., 2004) are among the important genomic data clarifying disease processes and medication success. This data allows tailored therapeutic recommendations to be created considering every patient's particular characteristics and medical history (Beam & Kohane, 2018). Deep learning algorithms developed by researchers examine the genetic and genomic traits of a tumor to forecast patient response to various chemotherapy drugs (Wang et al., 2022). By combining data on gene mutations, copy number variations, and epigenetic changes, these models can identify some biomarkers associated with therapy success. Integrating this data into the patient's optimal treatment plan may enhance the likelihood of a favorable outcome (Cuocolo et al., 2020). Deep learning algorithms use patient age medical history and surgery type alongside genomic information to calculate complication risks such as infections and hemorrhages. New monitoring techniques and preventive strategies for high-risk patients especially the impaired ones can lead to better outcomes by lowering complication rates. Persons with disabilities obtain substantial benefits from custom patient care when pharmacogenomic data creates precise medication dosing and identifies unsatisfactory drug reactions (McKillip et al., 2017).

Health professionals use genetic information through pharmacogenomics to optimize precision medicine by studying the way genetic variabilities affect therapeutic outcomes and side effects (Ryan et al., 2024). Pharmacogenomic information lets algorithms make predictions regarding the way a specific medication will affect each patient. Pharmacological concentration and therapeutic effects vary according to differences among transport proteins, drug targets, and metabolism enzymes (Wang et al., 2021). The use of pharmacogenomic data by AI models to identify individual patient-specific drug recommendations permits both superior therapeutic results and minimized medication side effects. The identification of individuals at risk for severe medicine side effects through pharmacogenomic information could result in more individualized treatment or prevention strategies. The analytical methodology offers patients safe medications which are specifically designed to match their genetic characteristics. Oncologists can improve hereditary illness patient treatment through pharmacist-genomic analysis to discover individualized pharmaceutical products (Varnai et al., 2019). Healthcare practitioners achieve better patient outcomes by implementing pharmacogenomic information into customized therapeutic choices.

5.4.4 *Predictive Models for Disease Progression and Risk Stratification*

Medical records analysis combined with genetic data alongside other relevant clinical information enables disease progression prediction models to estimate an individual with disability risks of acquiring specific illnesses and pre-existing condition deterioration. Medical models help doctors recognize people at elevated disease risk which allows physicians to establish preventative measures to lower their vulnerability to diseases (Cai et al., 2024). These models assist physicians in modifying treatment approaches when they provide probable patient disease progression information. The construction of predictive models depends on machine learning methods which process extensive patient data records. The analysis tools merge information about genetics and health records from patients to recognize possible disease indicators (López-Cortés et al., 2022). Healthcare providers enhance patient health outcomes when they use predictive models for disease progression and patient risk evaluation which allows them to develop preventive strategies and adjust treatment approaches (Mohsin et al., 2023). The algorithms possess the ability to determine disease progression levels while detecting individuals that are most likely to develop existing illnesses.

Multiple evaluation and forecasting methods have been created for illness probability assessment. The development of deep learning prediction models allows scientists to monitor Alzheimer's disease development through MRI brain scans combined with patient secondary information. Doctors use assessments to monitor the disease progression which helps them adjust the course of treatment. Prediction algorithms for cardiovascular disease evaluate patient heart condition risk by analyzing their genetics and measuring blood pressure alongside cholesterol results (D'Agostino et al., 2008). The gathered patient data helps clinicians become more efficient at recognizing at-risk patients so they can initiate early prevention actions. Predicting risk models utilizing patient data points consisting of genetics together with habits and ancestral lineage helps physicians identify at-risk cancer patients to administer preventive treatments before cancer onset (Zheng et al., 2022). Medical risk prediction tools for surgical complications evaluate a patient's chance of postoperative complications by combining data from patient features including their age surgical procedure and medical history (Zeng et al., 2021). Risk prediction through these methods provides hospitals with the capacity to detect patients that face greater complications enabling them to provide additional care for vulnerability mitigation. The readmission risk assessment algorithms analyze medical history data and age and sickness severity to determine readmission probabilities. Further monitoring of readmission-risk patients becomes possible when healthcare practitioners administer drugs or augment patient observation through the use of this approach (Costa et al., 2022). Deep learning models continue to spread through the healthcare industry because scientists predict these models will enhance both medical care quality and clinical results.

Medical treatments heavily rely on predictive models for both risk assessment in patients and disease progression tracking. Medical staff can utilize this skill to identify disabled patients that face higher risks of particular health conditions thus preparing suitable interventions (Yarborough et al., 2022). The system offers value but suffers from major problems which include inaccurate forecast possibilities and mistrust about the validity of training information. Healthcare models require error-free training datasets alongside consistent performance assessments to detect hidden bias or errors affecting predictions (Yarborough et al., 2022). The application of these diagnostic tools should be handled wisely to stop patients from receiving inappropriate treatment because of sufficing predictions. Preventative models used in clinical work need regular assessment of their operation alongside a detailed investigation of their therapeutic advantages to support their proper implementation. The training data sets need to demonstrate precise population representation for the intended purpose (Wiberg, 2022). Thorough patient information integration of demographics along with genetic and environmental variables is necessary for disease prediction models which forecast disease onset and risk across all patients without considering distinctive historical or characteristic attributes (Wiberg, 2022). These models require strict oversight together with informed patient consent and adherence to the highest ethical standards to protect patient groups from exploitation or unjust treatment (Obermeyer & Emanuel, 2016).

5.4.5 *Appointment Scheduling and Reminders*

Healthcare providers, particularly those assisting individuals with disabilities, substantially benefit from automated appointment reminders and scheduling systems,

5.4 Personalized Healthcare Solutions

as they improve patient adherence and alleviate the burden on healthcare professionals (Werner et al., 2023). Researchers anticipate that as deep learning models improve their ability to assess large volumes of patient data, the use of automated systems for appointment scheduling and reminder alerts will increase in the healthcare industry. Automated appointment notifications and scheduling are crucial in healthcare. This enhances the probability that patients will adhere to their treatment regimens. Utilizing AI, particularly deep learning models, can significantly enhance the accuracy and customization of these procedures through the analysis of extensive patient data. Implementation of deep learning algorithms determines the best appointment hours through a review of medical data and analysis of previous consultation records combined with patient preference information. A thorough examination improves healthcare operations and results which ultimately leads to better patient care including those requiring mobility assistance because it reduces schedule changes and postponements. AI systems improve appointment scheduling by matching patient needs with doctor availability based on human-inaccessible patterns in patient scheduling activities.

The use of automated appointment notifications forms an essential part of AI-based appointment scheduling systems. By analyzing patient data, encompassing demographics, medical history, and previous responses to reminders, deep learning algorithms can identify the most effective personalized appointment reminder (Posadzki et al., 2016). This tailored approach decreases the frequency of missed appointments and enhances the probability that compromised patients will have timely treatment. AI may swiftly modify reminder strategies in response to patient feedback, enhancing their efficacy. AI-enabled appointment scheduling and reminders are accessible on platforms like as Vyasa, Zocdoc, and PatientPop. Utilizing historical schedules and medical records, these systems employ AI to evaluate patient data and recommend optimal appointment times. Personal reminders enhance the probability that patients will attend their appointments and receive necessary care. By optimizing the online appointment booking system and delivering automated reminders to patients, these AI technologies reduce the substantial strain on healthcare staff.

Patients utilizing automated reminder systems exhibit a higher likelihood of attending their scheduled appointments. Studies indicate that individuals are more inclined to attend their planned medical appointments when reminded by text messages (Bjørnholt et al., 2016). Recent research (Dombkowski et al., 2017) indicates that email reminders enhance vaccination rates and subsequent appointments. However, other challenges regarding compliance and motivation exist beyond reminder systems. Aspects include patients' trust in clinicians, their understanding of the healthcare system, and the effectiveness of medications that significantly influence patient's compliance with treatment regimens. Researchers anticipate that AI-driven automated scheduling and reminders will gain prominence in healthcare as deep learning models advance. This will result in improved patient outcomes and enhanced healthcare delivery efficiency.

5.5 Conclusion

The incorporation of artificial intelligence (AI) in tailored care for individuals with impairments represents a substantial transformation, greatly improving assistance and accessibility. AI-driven assistive technologies have progressed swiftly, integrating breakthroughs like virtual assistant chatbots, wearable devices, predictive analytics, personalized regimens, and automated systems. These technologies enhance care quality while empowering individuals with disabilities through customized support and promoting increased independence. AI-driven individualized assistive technologies encompass motion detection for improved accessibility and visual analysis for tailored support. Moreover, AI improves healthcare with virtual assistant chatbots for patient support and education, telemonitoring with wearable devices, predictive disease analytics for personalized therapy, and automated appointment scheduling. Utilizing AI's capabilities, assistive technologies are advancing, fostering a more inclusive and engaging support system. These developments facilitate individuals with impairments in overcoming daily problems more effectively, enhancing their quality of life and social engagement.

References

Abd Rahman, R., Omar, K., Noah, S. A., Danuri, M. S., & Al-Garadi, M. A. (2020). Application of machine learning methods in mental health detection: A systematic review. *IEEE Access, 8*, 183952–183964.

Aggarwal, A., Tam, C. C., Wu, D., Li, X., & Qiao, S. (2023). Artificial intelligence–based chatbots for promoting health behavioral changes: Systematic review. *Journal of Medical Internet Research, 25*, e40789.

Al-Dulaimi, J. A. (2021). *IoT System engineering approach using AI for managing safety products in healthcare and workplaces* (Doctoral dissertation, Brunel University London).

Badidi, E., Moumane, K., & El Ghazi, F. (2023, August 1). Opportunities, applications, and challenges of edge-AI enabled video analytics in smart cities: A systematic review. IEEE Access.

Beam, A. L., & Kohane, I. S. (2018). Big data and machine learning in health care. *JAMA, 319*(13), 1317–1318.

Bertagnolli, M. M., Anderson, B., Quina, A., & Piantadosi, S. (2020). The electronic health record as a clinical trials tool: Opportunities and challenges. *Clinical Trials, 17*(3), 237–242.

Bjørnholt, K., Christiansen, E., Atterman Stokholm, K., & Hvolby, A. (2016). The effect of daily small text message reminders for medicine compliance amongst young people connected with the outpatient department for child and adolescent psychiatry. A controlled and randomized investigation. *Nordic Journal of Psychiatry, 70*(4), 285–289.

Bryant, B. R., & Seok, S. (2017). Introduction to the special series: Technology and disabilities in education. *Assistive Technology, 29*(3), 121–122.

Cai, Y., Cai, Y. Q., Tang, L. Y., Wang, Y. H., Gong, M., Jing, T. C., Li, H. J., Li-Ling, J., Hu, W., Yin, Z., & Gong, D. X. (2024). Artificial intelligence in the risk prediction models of cardiovascular disease and development of an independent validation screening tool: A systematic review. *BMC Medicine, 22*(1), 56.

Caliwag, A., Angsanto, S. R., & Lim, W. (2018, July 3). Korean sign language translation using machine learning. In *2018 Tenth International Conference on Ubiquitous and Future Networks (ICUFN)* (pp. 826–828). IEEE.

References

Calvaresi, D., Eggenschwiler, S., Mualla, Y., Schumacher, M., & Calbimonte, J. P. (2023). Exploring agent-based chatbots: A systematic literature review. *Journal of Ambient Intelligence and Humanized Computing, 14*(8), 11207–11226.

Carter, D., Kolencik, J., & Cug, J. (2021). Smart internet of things-enabled mobile-based health monitoring systems and medical big data in COVID-19 telemedicine. *American Journal of Medical Research, 8*(1), 20–29.

Challa, N. (2023). Artificial intelligence for object detection and its metadata. *The International Journal of Artificial Intelligence and Machine Learning (IJAIML), 2*, 121–133.

Chang, C. H. (2015). Deep and shallow architecture of multilayer neural networks. *IEEE Transactions on Neural Networks and Learning Systems, 26*(10), 2477–2486.

Chen, M., & Decary, M. (2020, January). Artificial intelligence in healthcare: An essential guide for health leaders. In *Healthcare management forum 2020* (Vol. 33, No. 1, pp. 10–18). SAGE Publications.

Chopde, R. (2024). *Comparative analysis of AI facial recognition algorithms* (Doctoral dissertation, Vellore Institute of Technology, India).

Corso, M. P., Perez, F. L., Stefenon, S. F., Yow, K. C., García Ovejero, R., & Leithardt, V. R. (2021). Classification of contaminated insulators using k-nearest neighbors based on computer vision. *Computers, 10*(9), 112.

Costa, M. L., Mafra, A. C., Cendoroglo, M. S., Rodrigues, P. S., Ferreira, M. S., Studenski, S. A., & Franco, F. G. (2022). Development and validation of predictive model for long-term hospitalization, readmission, and in-hospital death of patients over 60 years old. *Einstein (São Paulo), 20*, eAO8012.

Cuocolo, R., Caruso, M., Perillo, T., Ugga, L., & Petretta, M. (2020). Machine learning in oncology: A clinical appraisal. *Cancer Letters, 481*, 55–62.

D'Agostino, R. B., Sr., Vasan, R. S., Pencina, M. J., Wolf, P. A., Cobain, M., Massaro, J. M., & Kannel, W. B. (2008). General cardiovascular risk profile for use in primary care: The framingham heart study. *Circulation, 117*(6), 743–753.

da Silva, L. D., Pereira, T. F., Leithardt, V. R., Seman, L. O., & Zeferino, C. A. (2020). Hybrid impedance-admittance control for upper limb exoskeleton using electromyography. *Applied Sciences, 10*(20), 7146.

de Paz Santana, J. F., & de la Iglesia, D. H. (2021). *New trends in disruptive technologies, tech ethics and artificial intelligence.*

Dick, S. (2024, Mar 1) Virtual confessions: Examining the clergy privilege's extension to artificially intelligent religious robots. Available at SSRN 4745527.

Dingli, A., & Fournier, K. S. (2017). Financial time series forecasting-a deep learning approach. *International Journal of Machine Learning and Computing, 7*(5), 118–122.

Dombkowski, K. J., Cowan, A. E., Reeves, S. L., Foley, M. R., & Dempsey, A. F. (2017). The impacts of email reminder/recall on adolescent influenza vaccination. *Vaccine, 35*(23), 3089–3095.

Fernandes, F., Stefenon, S. F., Seman, L. O., Nied, A., Ferreira, F. C., Subtil, M. C., Klaar, A. C., & Leithardt, V. R. (2022). Long short-term memory stacking model to predict the number of cases and deaths caused by COVID-19. *Journal of Intelligent & Fuzzy Systems, 42*(6), 6221–6234.

Ficocelli, M., & Nejat, G. (2012). The design of an interactive assistive kitchen system. *Assistive Technology, 24*(4), 246–258.

Frizzo Stefenon, S., Seman, L. O., Schutel Furtado Neto, C., Nied, A., Seganfredo, D. M., Garcia da Luz, F., Sabino, P. H., Torreblanca González, J., & Quietinho Leithardt, V. R. (2020). Electric field evaluation using the finite element method and proxy models for the design of stator slots in a permanent magnet synchronous motor. *Electronics, 9*(11), 1975.

Frizzo Stefenon, S., Kasburg, C., Nied, A., Rodrigues Klaar, A. C., Silva Ferreira, F. C., & Waldrigues Branco, N. (2020). Hybrid deep learning for power generation forecasting in active solar trackers. *IET Generation, Transmission & Distribution, 14*(23), 5667–5674.

Frizzo Stefenon, S., Silva, M. C., Bertol, D. W., Meyer, L. H., & Nied, A. (2019). Fault diagnosis of insulators from ultrasound detection using neural networks. *Journal of Intelligent & Fuzzy Systems, 37*(5), 6655–6664.

Frizzo Stefenon, S., Waldrigues Branco, N., Nied, A., Wildgrube Bertol, D., Cristian Finardi, E., Sartori, A., Henrique Meyer, L., & Bartnik Grebogi, R. (2020). Analysis of training techniques of ANN for classification of insulators in electrical power systems. *IET Generation, Transmission & Distribution, 14*(8), 1591–1597.

Frizzo Stefenon, S., Zanetti Freire, R., dos Santos Coelho, L., Meyer, L. H., Bartnik Grebogi, R., Gouvêa Buratto, W., & Nied, A. (2020). Electrical insulator fault forecasting based on a wavelet neuro-fuzzy system. *Energies, 13*(2), 484.

Fuadi, D. H., Novita, D., & Taufik, M. (2021, April 28). Socially assistive robot interaction by objects detection and face recognition on convolutional neural network for parental monitoring. In *2021 International Conference on Artificial Intelligence and Mechatronics Systems (AIMS)* (pp. 1–6). IEEE.

Hashi, A. O., Hashim, S. Z., & Asamah, A. B. (2024, July 2). A systematic review of hand gesture recognition: An update from 2018 to 2024. IEEE Access

He, T., & Lee, C. (2021). Evolving flexible sensors, wearable and implantable technologies towards BodyNET for advanced healthcare and reinforced life quality. *IEEE Open Journal of Circuits and Systems, 2*, 702–720.

Hrabovska, N., Kajati, E., & Zolotova, I. (2023). A validation study to confirm the accuracy of wearable devices based on health data analysis. *Electronics, 12*(11), 2536.

Jacob, S., Alagirisamy, M., Xi, C., Balasubramanian, V., Srinivasan, R., Parvathi, R., Jhanjhi, N. Z., & Islam, S. M. (2021). AI and IoT-enabled smart exoskeleton system for rehabilitation of paralyzed people in connected communities. *IEEE Access, 9*, 80340–80350.

Kasburg, C., & Stefenon, S. F. (2019). Deep learning for photovoltaic generation forecast in active solar trackers. *IEEE Latin America Transactions, 17*(12), 2013–2019.

Kaur, J., Khan, M. A., Iftikhar, M., Imran, M., & Haq, Q. E. (2021). Machine learning techniques for 5G and beyond. *IEEE Access, 13*(9), 23472–23478.

Kearney, K. T., Presenza, D., Saccà, F., & Wright, P. (2018, September 17). Key challenges for developing a Socially Assistive Robotic (SAR) solution for the health sector. In *2018 IEEE 23rd international workshop on computer aided modeling and design of communication links and networks (CAMAD)* (pp. 1–7). IEEE.

Kim, D. E., & Gofman, M. (2018, January 8). Comparison of shallow and deep neural networks for network intrusion detection. In *2018 IEEE 8th Annual Computing and Communication Workshop and Conference (CCWC)* (pp. 204–208). IEEE.

King, P., & Martínez, E. G. (2020). Robotic assistive technologies: Principles and practice. *IEEE Pulse, 11*(1), 27–28.

Kumar, S. A., & Brown, M. A. (2018, November 18). Spatio-temporal reasoning within a neural network framework for intelligent physical systems. In *2018 IEEE Symposium Series on Computational Intelligence (SSCI)* (pp. 274–280). IEEE.

Kurniawan, M. H., Handiyani, H., Nuraini, T., Hariyati, R. T., & Sutrisno, S. (2024). A systematic review of artificial intelligence-powered (AI-powered) chatbot intervention for managing chronic illness. *Annals of Medicine, 56*(1), 2302980.

Leithardt, V., Santos, D., Silva, L., Viel, F., Zeferino, C., & Silva, J. (2020). A solution for dynamic management of user profiles in IoT environments. *IEEE Latin America Transactions, 18*(07), 1193–1199.

Liu, Z., Sun, H. X., Zhang, Y. W., Li, Y. F., Zuo, J., Meng, Y., & Fang, F. D. (2004). Effect of SNPs in protein kinase Cz gene on gene expression in the reporter gene detection system. *World Journal of Gastroenterology: WJG, 10*(16), 2357.

Lopes, H., Pires, I. M., Sánchez San Blas, H., García-Ovejero, R., & Leithardt, V. (2020). PriADA: management and adaptation of information based on data privacy in public environments. *Computers, 9*(4), 77.

López-Cortés, X. A., Matamala, F., Venegas, B., & Rivera, C. (2022). Machine-learning applications in oral cancer: A systematic review. *Applied Sciences, 12*(11), 5715.

Magalhaes Azevedo, D., & Kieffer, S. (2021). User reception of AI-enabled mHealth Apps: The case of Babylon health.

References

Marechal, C., Mikolajewski, D., Tyburek, K., Prokopowicz, P., Bougueroua, L., Ancourt, C., & Wegrzyn-Wolska, K. (2019). Survey on AI-based multimodal methods for emotion detection. *High-Performance Modelling and Simulation for Big Data Applications, 11400*, 307–324.

McKillip, R. P., Borden, B. A., Galecki, P., Ham, S. A., Patrick-Miller, L., Hall, J. P., Hussain, S., Danahey, K., Siegler, M., Sorrentino, M. J., & Sacro, Y. (2017). Patient perceptions of care as influenced by a large institutional pharmacogenomic implementation program. *Clinical Pharmacology & Therapeutics, 102*(1), 106–114.

Mohsin, S. N., Gapizov, A., Ekhator, C., Ain, N. U., Ahmad, S., Khan, M., Barker, C., Hussain, M., Malineni, J., Ramadhan, A., & Nagaraj, R. H. (2023). The role of artificial intelligence in prediction, risk stratification, and personalized treatment planning for congenital heart diseases. *Cureus, 15*(8).

Mora, N., Grossi, F., Russo, D., Barsocchi, P., Hu, R., Brunschwiler, T., Michel, B., Cocchi, F., Montanari, E., Nunziata, S., & Matrella, G. (2019). Iot-based home monitoring: Supporting practitioners' assessment by behavioral analysis. *Sensors, 19*(14), 3238.

Mukkamala, R., Yavarimanesh, M., Natarajan, K., Hahn, J. O., Kyriakoulis, K. G., Avolio, A. P., & Stergiou, G. S. (2021). Evaluation of the accuracy of cuffless blood pressure measurement devices: Challenges and proposals. *Hypertension, 78*(5), 1161–1167.

Nasr, M., Islam, M. M., Shehata, S., Karray, F., & Quintana, Y. (2021). Smart healthcare in the age of AI: Recent advances, challenges, and future prospects. *IEEE Access, 8*(9), 145248–145270.

Nguyen, T. N., Piuri, V., Qi, L., Mumtaz, S., & Lee, W. H. (2023). Guest editorial innovations in wearable, implantable, mobile, & remote healthcare with IoT & sensor informatics and patient monitoring. *IEEE Journal of Biomedical and Health Informatics, 27*(5), 2152–2154.

Ninno Muniz, R., Frizzo Stefenon, S., Gouvêa Buratto, W., Nied, A., Meyer, L. H., Finardi, E. C., Marino Kühl, R., Silva de Sa, J. A., & Ramati Pereira da Rocha, B. (2020). Tools for measuring energy sustainability: A comparative review. *Energies, 13*(9), 2366.

Obermeyer, Z., & Emanuel, E. J. (2016). Predicting the future—Big data, machine learning, and clinical medicine. *New England Journal of Medicine, 375*(13), 1216–1219.

Pinto, H. S., Américo, J. P., Leal, O. E., & Stefenon, S. F. (2021). Development of measurement device and data acquisition for electric vehicle. *Revista Geintec, 11*(1), 5809–5822.

Polyakov, E. V., Mazhanov, M. S., Rolich, A. Y., Voskov, L. S., Kachalova, M. V., & Polyakov, S. V. (2018, March 14). Investigation and development of the intelligent voice assistant for the Internet of Things using machine learning. In *2018 Moscow workshop on electronic and networking technologies (MWENT)* (pp. 1–5). IEEE.

Posadzki, P., Mastellos, N., Ryan, R., Gunn, L. H., Felix, L. M., Pappas, Y., Gagnon, M. P., Julious, S. A., Xiang, L., Oldenburg, B., & Car, J. (2016). Automated telephone communication systems for preventive healthcare and management of long-term conditions. *Cochrane Database of Systematic Reviews* (12).

Qian, K., Zhang, Z., Yamamoto, Y., & Schuller, B. W. (2021). Artificial intelligence internet of things for the elderly: From assisted living to health-care monitoring. *IEEE Signal Processing Magazine., 38*(4), 78–88.

Ryan, D. K., Maclean, R. H., Balston, A., Scourfield, A., Shah, A. D., & Ross, J. (2024). Artificial intelligence and machine learning for clinical pharmacology. *British Journal of Clinical Pharmacology, 90*(3), 629–639.

Sahoo, S. K., & Choudhury, B. B. (2023). AI advances in wheelchair navigation and control: A comprehensive review. *Journal of Process Management and New Technologies, 11*(3–4), 115–132.

Saini, R., Budhiraja, A., & Singh, S. (2024, February 16). Enhancing accessibility for the visually impaired: A multimodal approach. In *NIELIT's International Conference on Communication, Electronics and Digital Technologies* (pp. 457–470). Springer Nature Singapore.

Salazar, L. H., Fernandes, A., Dazzi, R., Garcia, N., & Leithardt, V. R. (2020). Using different models of machine learning to predict attendance at medical appointments. *Journal of Information Systems Engineering and Management, 5*(4), em0122.

Salazar, L. H., Fernandes, A. M., Dazzi, R., Raduenz, J., Garcia, N. M., & Leithardt, V. R. (2020, June 24) Prediction of attendance at medical appointments based on machine learning. In *2020 15th Iberian Conference on Information Systems and Technologies (CISTI)* (pp. 1–6). IEEE.

Salazar, L. H., Leithardt, V. R., Parreira, W. D., da Rocha Fernandes, A. M., Barbosa, J. L., & Correia, S. D. (2021). Application of machine learning techniques to predict a patient's no-show in the healthcare sector. *Future Internet, 14*(1), 3.

Sarkar, P. P., Tohin, M. A., Khaled, M. A., & Islam, M. R. (2019, November 29). Design process of an affordable smart robotic crutch for paralyzed patients. In *2019 IEEE International Conference on Robotics, Automation, Artificial-intelligence and Internet-of-Things (RAAICON)* (pp. 112–115). IEEE.

Sharma, R., Gandhi, K. R., Shanmugaraja, K., Sungheetha, A., Chinnaiyan, R., & Jegan, J. (2024, February 21). Motion detection using heuristic AI based machine learning approaches. In *2024 4th International Conference on Innovative Practices in Technology and Management (ICIPTM)* (pp. 1–4). IEEE.

Silva de Lima, A. L., Evers, L. J., Hahn, T., Bataille, L., Hamilton, J. L., Little, M. A., Okuma, Y., Bloem, B. R., & Faber, M. J. (2017). Freezing of gait and fall detection in Parkinson's disease using wearable sensors: A systematic review. *Journal of Neurology, 264*, 1642–1654.

Silva, L. A., Leithardt, V. R., Rolim, C. O., González, G. V., Geyer, C. F., & Silva, J. S. (2019). PRISER: Managing notification in multiples devices with data privacy support. *Sensors, 19*(14), 3098.

Soma, S., Patil, N., Salva, F., & Jadhav, V. (2018, July 10). An approach to develop a smart and intelligent wheelchair. In *2018 9th International Conference on Computing, Communication and Networking Technologies (ICCCNT)* (pp. 1–7). IEEE.

Sopelsa Neto, N. F., Stefenon, S. F., Meyer, L. H., Bruns, R., Nied, A., Seman, L. O., Gonzalez, G. V., Leithardt, V. R., & Yow, K. C. (2021). A study of multilayer perceptron networks applied to classification of ceramic insulators using ultrasound. *Applied Sciences, 11*(4), 1592.

Stefenon, S. F., Bruns, R., Sartori, A., Meyer, L. H., Ovejero, R. G., & Leithardt, V. R. (2022). Analysis of the ultrasonic signal in polymeric contaminated insulators through ensemble learning methods. *IEEE Access, 10*, 33980–33991.

Stefenon, S. F., Furtado Neto, C. S., Coelho, T. S., Nied, A., Yamaguchi, C. K., & Yow, K. C. (2022). Particle swarm optimization for design of insulators of distribution power system based on finite element method. *Electrical Engineering, 104*(2), 615–622.

Stefenon, S. F., Kasburg, C., Freire, R. Z., Silva Ferreira, F. C., Bertol, D. W., & Nied, A. (2021). Photovoltaic power forecasting using wavelet neuro-fuzzy for active solar trackers. *Journal of Intelligent & Fuzzy Systems, 40*(1), 1083–1096.

Stefenon, S. F., Ribeiro, M. H., Nied, A., Mariani, V. C., Coelho, L. D., Leithardt, V. R., Silva, L. A., & Seman, L. O. (2021). Hybrid wavelet stacking ensemble model for insulators contamination forecasting. *IEEE Access, 9*, 66387–66397.

Stefenon, S. F., Ribeiro, M. H., Nied, A., Mariani, V. C., dos Santos, C. L., da Rocha, D. F., Grebogi, R. B., & de Barros Ruano, A. E. (2020). Wavelet group method of data handling for fault prediction in electrical power insulators. *International Journal of Electrical Power & Energy Systems, 123*, 106269.

Stefenon, S. F., Ribeiro, M. H., Nied, A., Yow, K. C., Mariani, V. C., dos Santos, C. L., & Seman, L. O. (2022). Time series forecasting using ensemble learning methods for emergency prevention in hydroelectric power plants with dam. *Electric Power Systems Research, 202*, 107584.

Stefenon, S. F., Seman, L. O., Pavan, B. A., Ovejero, R. G., & Leithardt, V. R. (2022). Optimal design of electrical power distribution grid spacers using finite element method. *IET Generation, Transmission & Distribution, 16*(9), 1865–1876.

Sung, T. W., Tsai, P. W., Gaber, T., & Lee, C. Y. (2021, August 11). Artificial Intelligence of Things (AIoT) technologies and applications. *Wireless Communications and Mobile Computing*.

Tissot, H. C., Shah, A. D., Brealey, D., Harris, S., Agbakoba, R., Folarin, A., Romao, L., Roguski, L., Dobson, R., & Asselbergs, F. W. (2020). Natural language processing for mimicking clinical trial recruitment in critical care: A semi-automated simulation based on the LeoPARDS trial. *IEEE Journal of Biomedical and Health Informatics, 24*(10), 2950–2959.

Turing, A. M. (2009). *Computing machinery and intelligence*. Springer.

Varnai, R., Koskinen, L. M., Mäntylä, L. E., Szabo, I., FitzGerald, L. M., & Sipeky, C. (2019). Pharmacogenomic biomarkers in docetaxel treatment of prostate cancer: From discovery to implementation. *Genes, 10*(8), 599.

Vieira, J. C., Sartori, A., Stefenon, S. F., Perez, F. L., De Jesus, G. S., & Leithardt, V. R. (2022). Low-cost CNN for automatic violence recognition on embedded system. *IEEE Access, 10*, 25190–25202.

Viel, F., Silva, L. A., Leithardt, R. V., & Zeferino, C. A. (2018, November 12). Internet of Things: Concepts, architectures and technologies. In *2018 13th IEEE International Conference on Industry Applications (INDUSCON)* (pp. 909–916). IEEE.

Wang, Y., Yang, Y., Chen, S., & Wang, J. (2021). DeepDRK: A deep learning framework for drug repurposing through kernel-based multi-omics integration. *Briefings in Bioinformatics, 22*(5), bbab048.

Wang, C. W., Khalil, M. A., & Firdi, N. P. (2022). A survey on deep learning for precision oncology. *Diagnostics, 12*(6), 1489.

Wang, T. L., Wu, H. Y., Wang, W. Y., Chen, C. W., Chien, W. C., Chu, C. M., & Wu, Y. S. (2023). Assessment of heart rate monitoring during exercise with smart wristbands and a heart rhythm patch: Validation and comparison study. *JMIR Formative Research, 7*(1), e52519.

Werner, K., Alsuhaibani, S. A., Alsukait, R. F., Alshehri, R., Herbst, C. H., Alhajji, M., & Lin, T. K. (2023). Behavioural economic interventions to reduce health care appointment non-attendance: A systematic review and meta-analysis. *BMC Health Services Research, 23*(1), 1136.

Wiberg, H. M. (2022). *Data-driven healthcare via constraint learning and analytics* (Doctoral dissertation, Massachusetts Institute of Technology).

World Health Organization. (2011). World report on disability. World Health Organization.

Yarborough, B. J., Stumbo, S. P., Schneider, J., Richards, J. E., Hooker, S. A., & Rossom, R. (2022). Clinical implementation of suicide risk prediction models in healthcare: A qualitative study. *BMC Psychiatry, 22*(1), 789.

You, Y., Tsai, C. H., Li, Y., Ma, F., Heron, C., & Gui, X. (2023). Beyond self-diagnosis: How a chatbot-based symptom checker should respond. *ACM Transactions on Computer-Human Interaction, 30*(4), 1–44.

Zamani, E. D., Smyth, C., Gupta, S., & Dennehy, D. (2023). Artificial intelligence and big data analytics for supply chain resilience: A systematic literature review. *Annals of Operations Research, 327*(2), 605–632.

Zeng, S., Li, L., Hu, Y., Luo, L., & Fang, Y. (2021). Machine learning approaches for the prediction of postoperative complication risk in liver resection patients. *BMC Medical Informatics and Decision Making, 21*, 1.

Zhang, J., & Tao, D. (2020). Empowering things with intelligence: A survey of the progress, challenges, and opportunities in artificial intelligence of things. *IEEE Internet of Things Journal, 8*(10), 7789–7817.

Zheng, Y., Li, J., Wu, Z., Li, H., Cao, M., Li, N., & He, J. (2022). Risk prediction models for breast cancer: A systematic review. *British Medical Journal Open, 12*(7), e055398.

Zhou, H., Yang, Y., Ning, S., Liu, Z., Lang, C., Lin, Y., & Huang, D. (2018). Combining context and knowledge representations for chemical-disease relation extraction. *IEEE/ACM Transactions on Computational Biology and Bioinformatics, 16*(6), 1879–1889.

Zikky, M., Hakkun, R. Y., Rizqi, A. F., Hamid, A., Basuki, A. (2017, November 15). Development of educational game for recognizing Indonesian sign language (SIBI) and breaking down the communication barrier with deaf people. In *2017 21st International Computer Science and Engineering Conference (ICSEC)* (pp. 1–6). IEEE.

Chapter 6
AI to Empower People with Disabilities Communication and Autonomy

Abstract Individuals with linguistic or cognitive disabilities may have significant challenges in communication, frequently limiting their educational, social, and professional prospects. Artificial intelligence can empower those with impairments by improving communication and promoting increased autonomy. This chapter explores the way AI-driven devices aid those with disabilities via gesture detection, emotion recognition, and text recognition, facilitating enhanced connection. Furthermore, it explores sophisticated augmentative and alternative communication (AAC) systems, such as the Picture Exchange Communication System, recorded voice devices, and electronic tablet speech programs, which offer crucial assistance for non-verbal individuals. The chapter additionally explores AI-driven communication technology tailored for students with impairments, including AI-powered chatbots, communication help tools, facial expression analysis, and interactive robots. Utilizing AI's capabilities, these technologies improve accessibility and inclusion, enabling those with disabilities to participate more successfully in schooling, social interactions, and professional settings, therefore, enhancing their overall quality of life.

Keywords Autonomy · Communication · Augmentative and alternative communication · AI-driven assistive devices · Gesture recognition

6.1 Introduction

Communication, characterized by the capacity to engage with others, exchange ideas and information, and acquire knowledge, has become essential to contemporary existence. Individuals with impairments, especially deaf or mute persons, may have considerable obstacles in communication within social and professional environments when employing conventional methods (ZainEldin et al., 2024). A recent increase in demand for a more accessible and inclusive communication solution has emerged to address the different needs of this community. Artificial intelligence (AI) is enhancing the lives of those with disabilities by fostering enhanced communication and promoting increased autonomy. Artificial intelligence-driven assistive technology is eliminating obstacles, enabling those with mobility or speech impairments to communicate and engage more comprehensively in society. The integration of voice recognition technology, text-to-speech devices, and AI-driven eye-tracking software enables users to articulate their objectives with clarity (Almufareh et al., 2024). These enhancements foster a greater sense of inclusion in academic, professional, and personal spheres.

The utilization of AI facilitates greater self-sufficiency for individuals with disabilities. Smart home technology developed through AI enables users to manage their home lighting appliances and entry points with voice commands as well as hand gestures which secures both access and residence security (Varun et al., 2021). Wearable AI devices provide transcription and environment description benefits to people with visual and auditory handicaps. Machine learning algorithms revolutionize customized rehabilitation and education delivery by customizing learning solutions to meet individual student needs and boosting their capacity to acquire new capabilities per a recent study (Nahavandi et al., 2022). Researchers have extensively studied AI-based real-time communication systems specifically for disabled populations due to the complex nature of the technological field.

Professionals within this field actively work on developing creative solutions to help their impaired patients overcome communication barriers. Professionals in the field work toward implementing deep learning and artificial intelligence (AI) together with convolutional neural networks (CNNs) in their systems. Artificial intelligence provides substantial potential for sign language translation as well as improved natural communication ability among individuals who are hard of hearing or suffer speech disabilities (Strobel et al., 2023). Artificial intelligence technology advances create spaces that respect human autonomy and produce interactive relationships between users. Artificial intelligence generates an unrestricted environment which produces personalized solutions for multiple needs.

6.2 Communication Support

Modern artificial intelligence technology enhances comprehensive communication approaches which remove obstacles for people experiencing disabilities. AI-based communication technologies enable support for a diverse range of disabilities which affect hearing mobility and speech abilities. Through the use of speech-to-text and text-to-speech programs, people with hearing impairments can maintain communication through real-time transcription functionalities. The combination of augmentative communication devices with AI-driven voice assistants delivers effective speech communication to persons having difficulties in speaking (Mahmoudi-Dehaki et al., 2025). Artificial intelligence offers a benefit for people with disabilities through its power to boost their speaking and non-speech communication skills (Scassellati et al., 2018). The teaching of communication skills through independent practice sessions represents an effective technique which specifically targets the social development of students. The main means of communication involved sign language. The research investigated the way people with cognitive disabilities used Kinect v2 to develop their sign language communication Understanding (Gomez-Donoso et al., 2016). People with disabilities used this technology to link communication efforts with both robotic systems and human operators. The implementation of gesture recognition systems text recognition systems and emotion detection systems allowed researchers to create tools which helped people with disabilities communicate more easily.

The combination of artificial intelligence eye-tracking devices along with brain-computer interfaces provides people with mobility limitations the ability to operate digital systems through visual contact or mental image of machine operation (Barsan-Pipu, 2019). The learning capabilities of algorithms enable them to learn user-specific speech and hand gestures which becomes a foundation for creating customized communication systems. Device solutions for mental state analysis through gesture recognition together with text recognition and emotion recognition systems enhance connection efficiency (Al-Shamayleh et al., 2018). Such technologies let disabled individuals experience context-sensitive interactions which solve major communication problems. These instruments provide increased accessibility which allows users to achieve independence together with social inclusion. This section provides an extensive review of disability-enhancing technologies that improve accessibility for people with disabilities across their personal lives work environments and social interactions as well as their effect on specialized communication tools. The next section provides an in-depth analysis of these assistive communication devices.

6.2.1 Gesture Recognition

AI-driven gesture detection technologies alongside innovative systems help people with disabilities improve their environmental interaction through better communication along with increased autonomy (Fig. 6.1) (Almufareh et al., 2024). People facing mobility issues can benefit from sophisticated computer vision algorithms to operate their assistive devices through which they achieve enhanced capabilities for interactive functions. Waving your hand or making a fist offers an effective command of equipment and messaging systems to help people regain independence (Saborío-Taylor & Rojas-Ramírez, 2024). AI technology enables gesture recognition to convert signs along with other non-verbal gestures into operational commands (Han et al., 2024). The innovation establishes accessible ways for hard of hearing and completely deaf people to connect with others thereby supporting their involvement in present-day society. Utilizing natural hand movements provides users easier access to wheelchairs as well as computers and prosthetic limbs which simplifies the tasks of navigation and completion (Mohamed, 2024).

The use of gesture recognition technology enhanced by AI operates effectively for rehabilitation therapy and communication tools (Sahoo & Choudhury, 2024). Executive staff can track patients recovering from accidents or strokes through motion-tracking feedback to help restore full movement abilities (Senadheera et al., 2024).

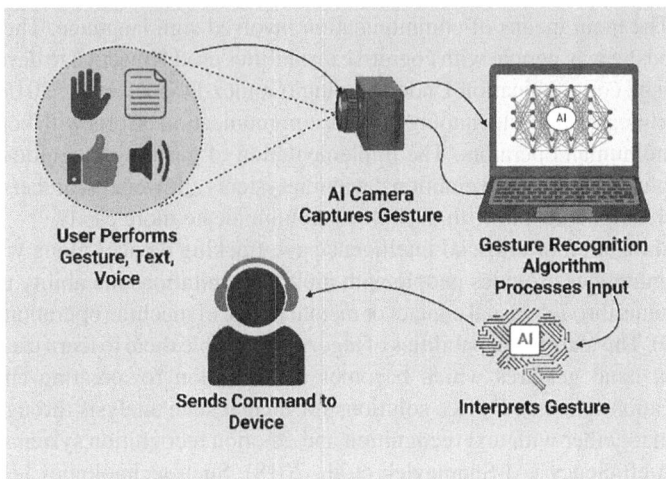

Fig. 6.1 Flowchart depicting an AI-driven gesture, image, text, and voice recognition system for individuals with disabilities, highlighting the natural transition from user-executed motions to device management via AI algorithms

Environmental control functions are possible through this technology which enables users to execute actions including door opening temperature adjustment and lighting modifications using hand movements. It facilitates their ability to manage their surroundings independently. AI-powered gesture recognition enhances communication and mobility through a natural, intuitive interface, promoting greater autonomy and inclusion, thereby improving the lives of those with disabilities.

6.2.2 Text Recognition

AI-driven computer vision algorithms are enhancing accessibility for individuals with disabilities by enabling the recognition and comprehension of text (Fig. 6.1) (Patel et al., 2025). These algorithms facilitate access to written information for those with visual impairments by converting printed text into audio or Braille formats. AI-enabled text recognition systems allow blind or visually impaired individuals to access the same information as sighted individuals, thereby eliminating obstacles in communication and daily activities (Chemnad & Othman, 2024). The AI reading assistance tool transforms picture and video texts into audio and Braille formats that help users understand essential information like menu items medical labels and building signs (Michalak & Ellixson, 2025). Document scanning enables text digitization for printed materials including books or articles which means users obtain content through speech or Braille formats. Users can view digital writings in text-based format on screens which allows them to customize font styles and benefits people with different accessibility needs.

6.2 Communication Support

People struggling with typing get help from AI-powered text recognition because it offers user-friendly text entry systems (Khamaj, 2025). Users can turn paper and screen texts into data entries for computers through interpretation processes. Through self-operating technology, AI generates video subtitles which boost accessibility for people with hearing difficulties. The AI technology enables visually impaired users to manage public spaces through automatic identification of signs labels and directions which include store names and bus numbers (Xie et al., 2022). Artificial intelligence (AI) text recognition constitutes a transformative force which promotes independence and societal inclusivity for people with disabilities because it eliminates communication barriers and information accessibility issues.

6.2.3 Emotion Recognition

The revolution of assistive technologies occurs through AI-driven computer vision algorithms. These algorithms analyze the emotional expressions of individuals as well as their vocal range and non-verbal signs to provide tailored assistance to users. Users can use emotion recognition systems to handle their anxiety and stress through emotion detection which triggers relaxation programs and additional support systems (Almufareh et al., 2024). This technology shows clear promise to improve disability-oriented communication while also providing better mental health care services education opportunities and social contact for patients. Emotion detection serves people with speech limitations through facial recognition and observation of body language (Kalateh et al., 2024). Open communication along with increased empathy becomes possible through technology which exposes a user's current emotional state to others. The ability to detect mood shifts based on voice tone variations together with altered facial expressions makes this tool valuable for mental health assessments. People along with healthcare providers gain the ability to quicken responses to developing mental health issues.

AI emotion recognition systems provide educational advantages combined with social feedback because they identify emotional states from both users and their surroundings (Shi, 2025). The technology helps users improve themselves and develop empathy by detecting emotional signals from voices and faces. The implementation of natural emotional input mechanisms leads users to better interact with assistive devices such as prosthetic limbs and voice recognition systems (Clark & Ahmad, 2023). Emotional identification improves through examining the social indicators like gestures and facial expressions which result in better social interactions by providing feedback about both intentions and emotions (Mehta et al., 2018). Through these capabilities, people can better interact with others to establish meaningful relationships. Assistive technology which employs AI-based emotion detection systems creates substantial enhancements to communication functions along with mental health support and education capabilities as well as improved social inclusion.

6.3 Augmentative and Alternative Communication (AAC)

People with impairments need augmentative and alternative communication (AAC) technology because it helps them communicate and remain engaged socially according to research (Mophosho & Masuku, 2021). The systems support a variety of user needs through picture exchange and recorded voice devices as well as electronic tablet speech apps. Recent technological improvements in artificial intelligence (AI) lead to enhanced AAC technology efficiency and customization which drives substantial changes in the industry. The integration of AI technology supports easier communication and diminishes physical requirements to fill communication gaps between users (Alam & Khan, 2024). The combination of NLP and ML algorithms enables e-speech applications to deliver context-based responses while they customize their operation according to user preferences and behaviors. This section investigates contemporary advances in augmentative and alternative communication (AAC) technology together with artificial intelligence methods which improve communication abilities for people with impairments and create inclusive systems that help users maintain independence in various settings.

6.3.1 Advanced AAC Systems

People having difficulties with verbal communication because of conditions like autism or cerebral palsy along with stroke or cancer often choose augmentative and alternative communication (AAC) devices to support their non-verbal communication (Donaldson et al., 2021). augmentative and alternative communication devices serve patients by providing brief immediacy aid in addition to long-term communication capabilities. The development of AAC systems by researchers led to the creation of both pictogram communication tools and limited vocabulary sentence generators (Donaldson et al., 2021). People struggling with motor control as well as vision difficulties and trouble processing information effectively learn to use pictogram-based augmentative communication devices. Specifically designed augmentative communication systems fit different users depending on critical attributes such as affordability and portable features, usage requirements, and efficiency during communication. The main categories of such systems incorporate electronic speech tablet applications with recorded speech devices and picture exchange communication systems.

The portable limitations and complex nature of inexpensive picture exchange communication tools which have extensive vocabulary act as their main drawbacks. Recorded voice devices are expensive yet have limited vocabulary but they provide both quick communication and portability (Beukelman & Mirenda, 1998). Electronic speech tablet applications maintain a perfect balance between their portability features and personalization options as well as their advanced features that include

6.3 Augmentative and Alternative Communication (AAC)

software updating capabilities and artificial intelligence components. The applications leverage AI through machine learning and natural language processing capabilities to create personalized user experiences and offer customizable communication features and improved communication effectiveness. Artificial intelligence (AI) based augmentative and alternative communication (AAC) platforms aid in improved communication along with social interaction for people with impairments through their ability to overcome communication challenges and supply authentic communication tools. The following section discusses methodology and advancement patterns in these transformative technologies.

6.3.1.1 Picture Exchange Communication System

Physical pictograms under the name Picture Exchange Communication (PEC) serve as core augmentative and alternative communication (AAC) technology to help disabled users express their wants and thoughts (Bondy & Frost, 1994). Users having multiple visual and cognitive abilities will receive the most benefit from implementing this technique. Managers should demonstrate well-developed motor skills to efficiently work with various pictograms at once. Multiple pictograms used in PEC systems make these systems cumbersome and difficult to move which presents a major drawback for these communication systems. High difficulty in locating particular pictograms decreases their effectiveness for fast communication because they hinder dynamic processes. Artificial intelligence solves these limitations by converting PEC systems into digital applications on mobile devices utilizing natural language processing and machine learning technologies (Talbott et al., 2015). The integrated system uses user behavior alongside context along with predictive pictogram suggestions to significantly decrease the time needed for searches. The application of AI makes PEC systems more portable and accessible leading to efficient user-friendly solutions that work across different situations and requirements.

The limitations of PEC systems do not hinder their broad use because they remain cost-efficient while numerous free resources remain accessible. The systems enable anyone to understand simple instructions while maintaining easy-to-use operation. The development of AI technologies is revolutionizing PEC systems through digital and mobile applications that utilize machine learning and natural language processing (Collet-Klingenberg, 2008). PEC systems experience improved accessibility and enhanced efficiency for people with impairments in various conditions through advances that promote user mobility along with automated pictogram selection and shortened communication times.

6.3.1.2 Recorded Speech Devices

People with communication problems can store speech of pre-programmed letters or sentences or phrases using Recorded Speech Devices (RSDs) (Emil et al., 2020). The

GoTalk Express 32 offers pictogram-based functionality to send multiple messages simultaneously while providing additional message cards as part of its operation (Emil et al., 2020). Engineers have designed these devices to work for mobile users through handle functionality and longer-lasting power. Users find pictogram-based Recorded Speech Devices easy to use because their limited selection of pre-programmed static choices improves communication effectiveness and enhances understanding. Users face delays when required messages do not appear on the currently active communication card since they must search and switch to different available pages. When a user needs food-related content but holds an animal-related card, they have to change cards which causes a delay in getting the desired message.

RSD systems work properly but their cost effectiveness varies between $165 and $700 and they do not support visual difficulty levels or motor skills or cognitive requirements (Kim & Ortega, 2023). The functionality of RSD systems receives improvement through artificial intelligence technology which enables users to personalize their voice while generating predictions for messages and adapting automatically to individual needs. The combination of machine learning (ML) with natural language processing (NLP) through artificial intelligence helps improve accessibility and reduces search durations and enhances message selection. Recent technological developments expand the range of communication possibilities because they enhance the functional capability and handheld convenience of RSDs for disabled users.

6.3.1.3 Electronic Tablet Speech Applications

An innovative category of pictogram-based Recorded Speech devices (RSDs) designed for smart devices such as tablets, smartwatches, and portable game consoles consists of electronic tablet speech applications. These applications enhance picture-to-speech functionalities by using the portability and processing capacity of contemporary smart devices, serving both academic and industrial purposes. Examples comprise Sc@ut (Rodríguez-Fórtiz et al., 2009), IMLIS (Schelhowe & Zare, 2009), Proloquo2Go (Lambright, 2023), Snap + Core First (Koerner et al., 2023), and Talk-Tablet (Radici et al., 2023). The dynamic pictogram exchange system is a significant feature of these applications. AAC applications utilize hierarchical folder systems to categorize pictograms meaningfully, unlike traditional RSDs. This arrangement enables users to swiftly locate the necessary options, facilitating expedited communication. Moreover, individuals with varying cognitive, visual, and motor capabilities can gain advantages from these applications, as they provide entirely personalized visual interfaces and tailored pictogram content.

Stratified learning methodologies enable products like Proloquo2Go to enhance creativity significantly. Starting with a fundamental collection of common terminology, users can progressively enhance their vocabulary and grammatical skills over time (Stone-MacDonald, 2015). The app prominently displays fundamental vocabulary on the main page. In topic-specific folders, infrequently utilized "fringe words" are also presented. The sophisticated functionalities enhance the versatility and user-friendliness of the communication tool. For instance, one can select the verb tense by pressing and holding a highlighted tile. Affordable pricing is another significant characteristic of AAC applications. For example, in comparison to other traditional RSDs, Proloquo2Go is a more economical option, priced at approximately $250. Smart gadgets provide users with easy portability because these solutions can be moved to any location. The reduced usability occurs when devices demand periodic charging during specific situations.

The software-powered system maintains up-to-date functionality and advanced technology capabilities as the leading advantage of electronic tablet speech applications. AI technologies specifically machine learning (ML) and natural language processing (NLP) serve as fundamental components which drive the evolution of these instruments. The interfaces of AI-driven AAC applications become customized and predict commonly used phrases and suitable pictograms because they monitor user behaviors and preferences (Akhtar & Rawol, 2024). Active electronic tablet speech programs currently serve as an effective solution for people with diverse disabilities because these devices reduce physical work and accelerate communication speed (Elsahar et al., 2019). The applications utilize AI capabilities to boost communication efficiency while users can benefit from their adaptable interface design which replaces conventional communication methods. Artificial intelligence (AI) significantly enhances independence and inclusion for those with communication impairments by integrating technology and accessibility.

6.4 AI Communication for Disabled Students

AI communication technologies are transforming education for children with impairments by providing accessible and customizable learning solutions (Habib et al., 2022). Individuals with auditory or verbal impairments can utilize voice-to-text and text-to-speech applications for seamless communication. Students with hearing impairments can enhance communication with voice assistants and AI-driven sign language recognition systems. Predictive text, alternative input devices, and AI-powered AAC (augmentative and alternative communication) systems support those with motor or cognitive impairments. Real-time translation and personalized learning platforms ensure inclusive education. By breaking communication barriers, AI fosters independence, engagement, and equal opportunities, empowering students with disabilities to learn and express themselves effectively. The next section explains the different applications of AI aiding communications for students with disability.

6.4.1 Adaptive Learning

Adaptive learning, facilitated by AI-driven communication technology, is enabling personalized and accessible educational experiences for students with disabilities (Fig. 6.2) (Strielkowski et al., 2024). These systems employ machine learning algorithms to evaluate student progress, adjust content delivery, and offer real-time individualized feedback.

The learning demands of students with learning disabilities are more varied than those of their peers without problems, resulting in increased obstacles in providing effective support for their education. The optimal instructional technique to address this difficulty is to offer tailored learning help or modify the educational materials to suit their requirements. The researcher developed an adaptive learning AI system aimed at a wide spectrum of ages, from under five years to adulthood, and accommodating various disorders, such as dyslexia and dysgraphia. Researchers have developed adaptive learning approaches utilizing AI to assist students with learning difficulties through intelligent serious games (Flogie et al., 2020), intelligent tutoring systems (Käser et al., 2013), and e-learning management systems (Alsobhi & Alyoubi, 2019). Researchers (Zingoni et al., 2021) created the BESPECIAL software platform to address the specific needs of dyslexic children by recognizing their challenges and offering tailored digital support strategies and educational materials. BESPECIAL develops its AI algorithms utilizing data obtained from students' clinical dyslexia reports, surveys, and psychometric assessments. The system can anticipate the needs of students with certain learning disabilities (such as memory impairments or focused attention challenges) and offer tailored adaptive solutions (such as concept maps, diagrams, or emphasized text) due to the implemented AI algorithms. Educators also acquire access to individualized tactics and optimal practices for

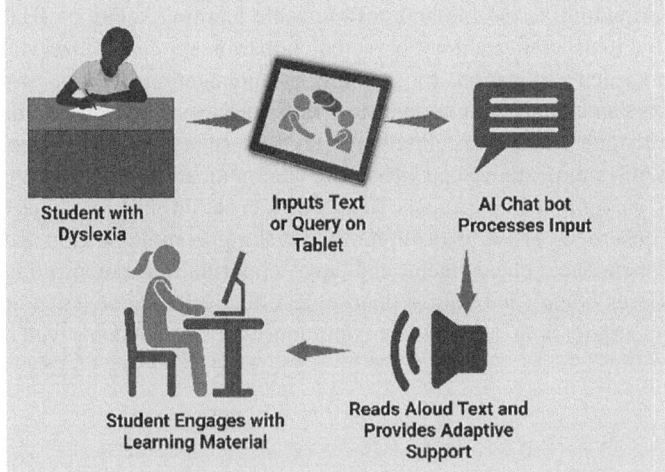

Fig. 6.2 Overview of AI-integrated adaptive learning for students with disabilities

students. Additionally, speech-to-text, text-to-speech, and gesture recognition tools enhance communication for those with speech, hearing, or mobility impairments. AI-powered chatbots and virtual assistants provide prompt support, fostering independence and engagement (Tahir & Tahir, 2023). Adaptive learning facilitates the academic success of children with disabilities by promoting an inclusive environment tailored to their unique learning styles. This enables individuals to surmount challenges and achieve academic success.

6.4.2 Facial Expression

Students with impairments are significantly benefiting from AI-powered facial expression detection by enhancing their ability to engage in learning and communication (Kushwaha, 2024). AI-driven systems analyze facial expressions to interpret emotions, helping educators tailor support based on students' needs. Active engagement of students in class is a crucial initial step in facilitating their learning, especially for those facing academic challenges. Research analysts detect student interest levels in education content by studying facial expressions. Researchers implemented artificial intelligence systems to evaluate facial expression data to forecast student information interaction levels. The evaluations of student facial expressions from ages 7 to 12 involved the utilization of support vector machines (Abdul Hamid et al., 2018) together with convolutional neural networks (CNN) (Hamid et al. 2018) and bag of features (BOF) (Ouherrou et al., 2019) and speed-up robust features (SURF) (Hamid et al., 2018) under artificial intelligence control. The first study measured SWLD content engagement through facial expression analysis that combined computer vision front face detection methods while the second study employed deep learning algorithms to detect subtle facial expression changes in students during learning activities. Educators gain important insights from facial analysis tools through student engagement assessments for students with learning disabilities and activity evaluation regarding student interest. Non-verbal students benefit from expression recognition because it creates better communication possibilities through responses that understand emotions (Alsaadawi et al., 2024). Integrated with adaptive learning platforms, these technologies personalize educational experiences, fostering inclusivity and emotional well-being. Artificial intelligence (AI) enhances student–teacher interaction by interpreting complex facial cues, fostering an inclusive classroom that adapts to each student's distinct requirements and promotes active engagement.

6.4.3 Chat Robot

With the growing prevalence of chatbots on digital platforms pertinent to students' life, numerous students globally have become acquainted with the use of chatbots or intelligent assistants due to technological advancements. Large corporations have employed chat robot AI technology for customer assistance and product troubleshooting, which has spurred its application in education. The chatbot can be employed to assist SWLDs (Rai et al., 2023). AI-powered chat robots are transforming education for disabled students by providing instant, accessible, and personalized learning support. These digital assistants offer students prompt response through explanations, reminders, and guidance by utilizing natural language processing (NLP) to analyze student inquiries (Antonius et al., 2023).

Sammy, an intelligent assistant utilized in a study, engaged with students over chat to furnish them with answers to their inquiries, referrals to pertinent resources, and tailored feedback (Gupta & Chen, 2022). A further study employed ALEXZA, a smartphone application, to assist individuals with dyslexia in reading through methods such as reading aloud, text chunking, and highlighting, among others (Rajapakse et al., 2018). The intelligent assistant within the application is capable of directly responding to user inquiries. Both researches employed an AI-powered chat assistant to offer accessibility assistance to students with reading-related learning difficulties. For students with speech or motor impairments, text-based or voice-activated chatbots facilitate seamless communication and interaction (Zaugg, 2024). Adaptive learning systems integrated with AI chatbots personalize instruction, ensuring that content is delivered in an accessible and engaging manner. By promoting independence, reducing learning barriers, and offering 24/7 support, AI chat robots empower disabled students to achieve scholarly achievement with greater ease.

6.4.4 Communication Assistant

SWLDs (Student with learning disabilities) encounter challenges in communication because of their inability to articulate thoughts verbally or in writing, which is exacerbated by an absence of confidence arising from their language-based difficulties. Communication aids can serve as valuable resources in facilitating interactions between students with learning disabilities and their peers and adults (Klefbeck, 2023). AI-powered communication assistants are revolutionizing support for students with disabilities by enhancing accessibility and interaction. These intelligent tools leverage speech-to-text, text-to-speech, and predictive text technologies to assist individuals with speech, hearing, or motor impairments in expressing themselves effectively (Latif et al., 2015). Researchers employed AI technology as a communicative aid to assist the disabled, particularly those with dyslexia. To assist students with voice communication, a researcher incorporated AI into an AAC gadget (Wang et al., 2022).

Real-time transcription, voice recognition, and emotion-aware AI enable seamless communication in both educational and social settings. In another work, researchers employed Neural Machine Translation (NMT) to create a tool named Additional Writing Help (AWH). This technology "translated" material exhibiting common dyslexic writing issues into a coherent format while preserving socially popular components such as slang, tags, hashtags, and mentions (Wu et al., 2019). Integrated with adaptive learning systems, communication assistants personalize interactions, fostering independence and confidence. By breaking down communication barriers, these AI-driven solutions enable students with impairments to participate more comprehensively in education, collaborate with peers, and navigate daily challenges with greater ease and efficiency (Mpia Ndombo et al., 2013).

6.4.5 Interactive Robot

AI-driven interactive robots are revolutionizing education for kids with disabilities by offering interesting, adaptive, and accessible learning opportunities. These robots use speech recognition, facial expression analysis, and gesture-based interactions to facilitate communication and personalized support. The social robot may physically engage with people with disabilities through the application of machine learning technologies. This study concentrated on assessing student engagement through the employment of an interactive robot, employed as an AI instrument to assist students with learning disabilities (Papakostas et al., 2021). The social robot, unlike the chatbot, engaged with SWLDs and employed multimodal machine learning to forecast their level of class participation (Sharif & Elmedany, 2022; Panjwani-Charania & Zhai, 2023). For students with autism, mobility impairments, or speech disorders, interactive robots serve as social and educational companions, enhancing engagement and learning through tailored responses. They promote engagement and independence by employing AI-driven adaptive learning technologies to adjust their teaching methods according to individuals' unique development. By fostering social interaction, improving cognitive skills, and offering real-time assistance, interactive robots empower students with disabilities to thrive in education.

6.5 Conclusion

In summary, AI-driven communication tools are revolutionizing the lives of individuals with verbal or cognitive disabilities by improving their capacity to interact and engage with their environment. AI enhances autonomy and accessibility for those with impairments through the utilization of gesture recognition, emotion recognition, and text recognition. Advanced augmentative and alternative communication (AAC) systems, such as the Picture Exchange Communication System, speech-generating devices, and electronic tablet applications, offer essential assistance for non-verbal individuals. Furthermore, AI-driven solutions including chatbots, communication assistance programs, facial expression analysis, and interactive robots are essential in supporting students with impairments in their educational pursuits. These innovations enhance communication and foster more inclusive educational, social, and professional contexts, guaranteeing equitable opportunity for all.

References

Abdul Hamid, S. S., Admodisastro, N., Manshor, N., Kamaruddin, A., & Ghani, A. A. (2018). Dyslexia adaptive learning model: Student engagement prediction using machine learning approach. In *Recent Advances on Soft Computing and Data Mining: Proceedings of the Third International Conference on Soft Computing and Data Mining (SCDM 2018), Johor, Malaysia, February 06–07, 2018* (pp. 372–384). Springer International Publishing.

Akhtar, Z. B., & Rawol, A. T. (2024). Enhancing cybersecurity through AI-powered security mechanisms. *IT Journal Research and Development, 9*(1), 50–67.

Alam, S., & Khan, M. F. (2024). Enhancing AI-human collaborative decision-making in industry 4.0 management practices. *IEEE Access*.

Almufareh, M. F., Kausar, S., Humayun, M., & Tehsin, S. (2024). A conceptual model for inclusive technology: Advancing disability inclusion through artificial intelligence. *Journal of Disability Research, 3*(1), 20230060.

Alsaadawi, H. F., Das, B., & Das, R. (2024). TAC-Trimodal Affective Computing: Principles, integration process, affective detection, challenges, and solutions. *Displays, 3*, 102731.

Al-Shamayleh, A. S., Ahmad, R., Abushariah, M. A., Alam, K. A., & Jomhari, N. (2018). A systematic literature review on vision based gesture recognition techniques. *Multimedia Tools and Applications, 77*, 28121–28184.

Alsobhi, A. Y., & Alyoubi, K. H. (2019). Adaptation algorithms for selecting personalised learning experience based on learning style and dyslexia type. *Data Technologies and Applications, 53*(2), 189–200.

Antonius, F., Alapati, P. R., Ritonga, M., Patra, I., El-Ebiary, Y. A., Orosoo, M., & Rengarajan, M. (2023). Incorporating natural language processing into virtual assistants: An intelligent assessment strategy for enhancing language comprehension. *International Journal of Advanced Computer Science and Applications, 14*(10).

Barsan-Pipu, C. (2020). Artificial intelligence applied to brain-computer interfacing with eye-tracking for computer-aided conceptual architectural design in virtual reality using neurofeedback. In *Proceedings of the 2019 DigitalFUTURES: The 1st International Conference on Computational Design and Robotic Fabrication (CDRF 2019)* (pp. 124–135). Springer.

Beukelman, D. R., & Mirenda, P. (1998). *Augmentative and alternative communication*. Paul H. Brookes.

Bondy, A. S., & Frost, L. A. (1994). The picture exchange communication system. *Focus on Autistic Behavior, 9*(3), 1–9.

Chemnad, K., & Othman, A. (2024). Digital accessibility in the era of artificial intelligence—Bibliometric analysis and systematic review. *Frontiers in Artificial Intelligence, 7*, 1349668.

Clark, A., & Ahmad, I. (2023). Touchless and nonverbal human-robot interfaces: An overview of the state-of-the-art. *Smart Health, 27*, 100365.

Collet-Klingenberg, L. (2008). *PECS: Steps for implementation*. The National Professional Development Center on Autism Spectrum Disorders, The Waisman Center, The University of Wisconsin.

References

Donaldson, A. L., corbin, E., & McCoy, J. (2021). "Everyone deserves AAC": Preliminary study of the experiences of speaking autistic adults who use augmentative and alternative communication. *Perspectives of the ASHA Special Interest Groups, 6*(2), 315–326.

Elsahar, Y., Hu, S., Bouazza-Marouf, K., Kerr, D., & Mansor, A. (2019). Augmentative and alternative communication (AAC) advances: A review of configurations for individuals with a speech disability. *Sensors, 19*(8), 1911.

Emil, Z., Robbertz, A., Valente, R., & Winsor, C. (2020). *Towards a more inclusive world: Enhanced augmentative and alternative communication for people with disabilities using ai and nlp*. Worcester Polytechnic Institute.

Flogie, A., Aberšek, B., Kordigel Aberšek, M., Sik Lanyi, C., & Pesek, I. (2020). Development and evaluation of intelligent serious games for children with learning difficulties: Observational study. *JMIR Serious Games, 8*(2), e13190.

Gomez-Donoso, F., Cazorla, M., Garcia-Garcia, A., & Garcia-Rodriguez, J. (2016). Automatic Schaeffer's gestures recognition system. *Expert Systems, 33*(5), 480–488.

Gupta, S., & Chen, Y. (2022). Supporting inclusive learning using chatbots? A chatbot-led interview study. *Journal of Information Systems Education, 33*(1), 98–108.

Habib, H., Jelani, S. A., & Najla, S. (2022). Revolutionizing Inclusion: AI in Adaptive Learning for Students with Disabilities. *Multidisciplinary Science Journal, 1*(01), 1–1.

Hamid, S. S., Admodisastro, N., Manshor, N., Ghani, A. A., & Kamaruddin, A. (2018, March 23). Engagement prediction in the adaptive learning model for students with dyslexia. In *Proceedings of the 4th International Conference on Human-Computer Interaction and User Experience in Indonesia, CHIuXiD'18* (pp. 66–73).

Han, L., Afzal, N., Wang, Z., Wang, Z., Jin, T., Guo, S., Gong, H., & Wang, D. (2024). Ambient haptics: Bilateral interaction among human, machines and virtual/real environments in pervasive computing era. *CCF Transactions on Pervasive Computing and Interaction, 4*, 1–33.

Kalateh, S., Estrada-Jimenez, L. A., Hojjati, S. N., & Barata, J. (2024). A systematic review on multimodal emotion recognition: Building blocks, current state, applications, and challenges. *IEEE Access*.

Käser, T., Busetto, A. G., Solenthaler, B., Baschera, G. M., Kohn, J., Kucian, K., von Aster, M., & Gross, M. (2013). Modelling and optimizing mathematics learning in children. *International Journal of Artificial Intelligence in Education, 23*, 115–35.

Khamaj, A. (2025). Ai-enhanced chatbot for improving healthcare usability and accessibility for older adults. *Alexandria Engineering Journal, 116*, 202–213.

Kim, J., & Ortega, N. (2023). Still finding their voice: For decades, assistive communication devices were available only to a small fraction of non-speaking people. The iPad should have revolutionized access. What happened? *MIT Technology Review, 126*(4), 42–50.

Klefbeck, K. (2023). Educational approaches to improve communication skills of learners with autism spectrum disorder and comorbid intellectual disability: An integrative systematic review. *Scandinavian Journal of Educational Research, 67*(1), 51–68.

Koerner, S. M., Glaser, S., & Kropkowski, K. (2023). Perspectives of part-time augmentative and alternative communication use in adults and implications for pediatric service delivery. *Perspectives of the ASHA Special Interest Groups, 8*(4), 747–760.

Kushwaha, A. (2024). AI and non-verbal communication: Enhancing understanding of emotional cues for hearing impairment children. *As the editors of Transforming Learning: The Power of Educational*, 13.

Lambright, N. L. (2023). Proloquo2Go (P2G) in the classroom: Providing speech, communication, behavioral support, academic, and social support for students. In *Using Assistive Technology for Inclusive Learning in K-12 Classrooms 2023* (pp. 140–155). IGI Global.

Latif, S., Tariq, R., Tariq, S., & Latif, R. (2015). Designing an assistive learning aid for writing acquisition: A challenge for children with dyslexia. In *Assistive technology* (pp. 180–188). IOS Press.

Mahmoudi-Dehaki, M., Nasr-Esfahani, N., & Vasan, S. (2025). The transformative role of assistive technology in enhancing quality of life for individuals with disabilities. In *Assistive technology solutions for aging adults and individuals with disabilities 2025* (pp. 45–72). IGI Global Scientific Publishing.

Mehta, D., Siddiqui, M. F., & Javaid, A. Y. (2018). Facial emotion recognition: A survey and real-world user experiences in mixed reality. *Sensors, 18*(2), 416.

Michalak, R., & Ellixson, D. (2025). Addressing language and ableism in information technology: A call to action for academic librarians. *Journal of Library Administration, 65*(1), 100–131.

Mohamed, N. (2024). Eye-gesture control of computer systems via artificial intelligence. *F1000Research, 13*, 109.

Mophosho, M., & Masuku, K. (2021, March 24). The uses of augmentative and alternative communication technology in empowering learners overcome communication barriers to learning. In *Empowering students and maximising inclusiveness and equality through ICT 2021* (pp. 203–222). Brill.

Mpia Ndombo, D., Ojo, S., & Osunmakinde, I. (2013). An intelligent integrative assistive system for dyslexic learners. *Journal of Assistive Technologies, 7*(3), 172–187.

Nahavandi, D., Alizadehsani, R., Khosravi, A., & Acharya, U. R. (2022). Application of artificial intelligence in wearable devices: Opportunities and challenges. *Computer Methods and Programs in Biomedicine, 213*, 106541.

Ouherrou, N., Elhammoumi, O., Benmarrakchi, F., & El Kafi, J. (2019). Comparative study on emotions analysis from facial expressions in children with and without learning disabilities in virtual learning environment. *Education and Information Technologies, 24*(2), 1777–92.

Panjwani-Charania, S., & Zhai, X. (2023). AI for students with learning disabilities: A systematic review.

Papakostas, G. A., Sidiropoulos, G. K., Lytridis, C., Bazinas, C., Kaburlasos, V. G., Kourampa, E., Karageorgiou, E., Kechayas, P., & Papadopoulou, M. T. (2021). Estimating children engagement interacting with robots in special education using machine learning. *Mathematical Problems in Engineering, 2021*(1), 9955212.

Patel, P., Pampaniya, S., Ghosh, A., Raj, R., Karuppaih, D., & Kandasamy, S. (2025). Enhancing accessibility through machine learning: A review on visual and hearing impairment technologies. *IEEE Access*.

Radici, E., Heboyan, V., & De Leo, G. (2023). A speech-to-symbol app for supporting communication partner to model and improve vocabulary. *Child Language Teaching and Therapy, 39*(3), 266–274.

Rai, H. L., Saluja, N., & Pimplapure, A. (2023). AI and learning disabilities: Ethical and social considerations in educational technology. *Educational Administration: Theory and Practice, 29*(4), 726–733.

Rajapakse, S., Polwattage, D., Guruge, U., Jayathilaka, I., Edirisinghe, T., & Thelijjagoda, S. (2018, December 5). ALEXZA: A mobile application for dyslexics utilizing artificial intelligence and machine learning concepts. In *2018 3rd International Conference on Information Technology Research (ICITR)* (pp. 1–6). IEEE.

Rodríguez-Fórtiz, M. J., González, J. L., Fernández, A., Entrena, M., Hornos, M. J., Pérez, A., Carrillo, A., & Barragán, L. (2009). Sc@ut: Developing adapted communicators for special education. *Procedia-Social and Behavioral Sciences, 1*(1), 1348–1352.

Saborío-Taylor, S., & Rojas-Ramírez, F. (2024). Universal design for learning and artificial intelligence in the digital era: Fostering inclusion and autonomous learning. *International Journal of Professional Development, Learners and Learning, 6*2.

Sahoo, S., & Choudhury, B. (2024). Exploring the use of computer vision in assistive technologies for individuals with disabilities: A review. *Journal of Future Sustainability, 4*(3), 133–48.

Scassellati, B., Boccanfuso, L., Huang, C. M., Mademtzi, M., Qin, M., Salomons, N., Ventola, P., & Shic, F. (2018). Improving social skills in children with ASD using a long-term, in-home social robot. *Science Robotics, 3*(21), eaat7544.

References

Schelhowe H, Zare S. Intelligent mobile interaction: a learning system for mentally disabled people (IMLIS). InUniversal Access in Human-Computer Interaction. Addressing Diversity: 5th International Conference, UAHCI 2009, Held as Part of HCI International 2009, San Diego, CA, USA, July 19–24 2009 Schelhowe, H., & Zare, S. (2009). Intelligent mobile interaction: A learning system for mentally disabled people (IMLIS). In *Universal Access in Human-Computer Interaction. Addressing Diversity: 5th International Conference, UAHCI 2009, Held as Part of HCI International 2009, San Diego, CA, USA, July 19-24, 2009. Proceedings, Part I 5 2009* (pp. 412–421). Springer.

Senadheera, I., Hettiarachchi, P., Haslam, B., Nawaratne, R., Sheehan, J., Lockwood, K. J., Alahakoon, D., & Carey, L. M. (2024). AI applications in adult stroke recovery and rehabilitation: A scoping review using AI. *Sensors (Basel, Switzerland), 24*(20), 6585.

Sharif, M. S., & Elmedany, W. (2022, March 28). A proposed machine learning based approach to support students with learning difficulties in the post-pandemic norm. In *2022 IEEE Global Engineering Education Conference (EDUCON)* (pp. 1988–1993). IEEE.

Shi, L. (2025). The integration of advanced AI-enabled emotion detection and adaptive learning systems for improved emotional regulation. *Journal of Educational Computing Research, 63*(1), 173–201.

Stone-MacDonald, A. (2015). Using iPad applications to increase literacy skills for children preK to grade 3 with disabilities. *Young Exceptional Children, 18*(3), 3–18.

Strielkowski, W., Grebennikova, V., Lisovskiy, A., Rakhimova, G., & Vasileva, T. (2024). AI-driven adaptive learning for sustainable educational transformation. *Sustainable Development*.

Strobel, G., Schoormann, T., Banh, L., & Möller, F. (2023). Artificial intelligence for sign language translation–A design science research study. *Communications of the Association for Information Systems, 53*(1), 22.

Tahir, A., & Tahir, A. (2023). AI-driven advancements in ESL learner autonomy: Investigating student attitudes towards virtual assistant usability. *Linguistic Forum-A Journal of Linguistics, 5*(2), 50–56.

Talbott, E. O., Marshall, L. P., Rager, J. R., Arena, V. C., Sharma, R. K., & Stacy, S. L. (2015). Air toxics and the risk of autism spectrum disorder: The results of a population based case–control study in southwestern Pennsylvania. *Environmental Health, 14*, 1–6.

Varun, A., Reddy, E. A., & Maheshwari, K. M. (2021). A smart home automation with personalised voice assistant using IOT. *Turkish Online Journal of Qualitative Inquiry, 12*(3).

Wang, M., Muthu, B., & Sivaparthipan, C. B. (2022). Smart assistance to dyslexia students using artificial intelligence based augmentative alternative communication. *International Journal of Speech Technology, 25*(2), 343–353.

Wu, S., Reynolds, L., Li, X., & Guzmán, F. (2019, May 2). Design and evaluation of a social media writing support tool for people with dyslexia. In *Proceedings of the 2019 CHI Conference on Human Factors in Computing Systems* (pp. 1–14).

Xie, J., Reddie, M., Lee, S., Billah, S. M., Zhou, Z., Tsai, C. H., & Carroll, J. M. (2022). Iterative design and prototyping of computer vision mediated remote sighted assistance. *ACM Transactions on Computer-Human Interaction (TOCHI), 29*(4), 1–40.

ZainEldin, H., Gamel, S. A., Talaat, F. M., Aljohani, M., Baghdadi, N. A., Malki, A., Badawy, M., & Elhosseini, M. A. (2024). Silent no more: A comprehensive review of artificial intelligence, deep learning, and machine learning in facilitating deaf and mute communication. *Artificial Intelligence Review, 57*(7), 188.

Zaugg, T. (2024). Future innovations for assistive technology and universal design for learning. In *Assistive technology and universal design for learning: Toolkits for inclusive instruction* (pp. 275–318).

Zingoni, A., Taborri, J., Panetti, V., Bonechi, S., Aparicio-Martínez, P., Pinzi, S., & Calabrò, G. (2021). Investigating issues and needs of dyslexic students at university: Proof of concept of an artificial intelligence and virtual reality-based supporting platform and preliminary results. *Applied Sciences, 11*(10), 4624.

Chapter 7
The Future of AI in Revolutionizing Support for Disabled Persons

Abstract Individuals with impairments have always encountered prejudice and marginalization stemming from societal assumptions regarding their capacities. Nonetheless, breakthroughs in AI are reshaping this narrative, providing robust solutions that improve both routine and intricate work. AI-driven technologies are dismantling obstacles, enhancing inclusion, and facilitating unprecedented autonomy. The future of AI-driven support possesses significant potential to transform assistance for individuals with disabilities in multiple areas, such as communication, education, and healthcare. This chapter examines the way AI tools will transform independence through facilitating seamless engagement, individualized education, and enhanced healthcare accessibility. Moreover, AI-enhanced smart home systems will augment convenience and safety, while AI-facilitated accessibility technologies will boost mobility and engagement for those with disabilities. The amalgamation of IoT with advanced AR/VR technologies will enhance assistive support, delivering immersive and intuitive experiences. This chapter also examines the future of autonomous cars tailored for those with disabilities, enhancing mobility and autonomy. These breakthroughs enable AI to transform the domain of disability support, fostering a more inclusive and accessible future.As keywords are mandatory for this chapter, please provide 3-6 keywords.Keywords: Augmented reality, Virtual reality, Education support, Healthcare, Smart homes

Keyword Augmented reality · Virtual reality · Education support · Healthcare · Smart homes

7.1 Introduction

Individuals with disabilities have historically encountered discrimination and exclusion stemming from the societal belief in their incapacity. Recently, there has been a notable change in this perception. Recent advancements in artificial intelligence hold the promise of transforming the future and experiences of individuals with disabilities by offering effective solutions that streamline both routine and intricate activities. The extensive application of AI leads to barrier elimination and creates inclusive opportunities that generate substantial autonomy levels (Olszewski et al., 2019; World Health Organization, 2019). In 2024, data given by the WHO (World Health Organisation) indicated that 1.5 billion individuals globally experience a notable disability. Statistically fifty million people globally experience deafness or low vision conditions accompanied by another fifty million people with vision impairments or blindness (Semary et al., 2024). Additionally, approximately 89% of individuals with disabilities reside in developing nations.

Artificial Intelligence has been creating new and more straightforward methods for managing everyday life. AI technology shows great potential for automating previously manual work functions that include visual perception together with voice recognition decision-support systems and predictive text generation. People with impairments receive substantial help from this technology to navigate their surroundings and carry out daily tasks. Visual assistance stands as an advanced Augmentative and alternative communication (AAC) approach which enables severe communicational disabilities in people across the globe to interact better with their environments (Light et al., 2019). The ability to participate in social settings together with communication, education, and work becomes impossible whenever these communication aids are removed (Schreibman et al., 2015). Individuals with impairments encounter challenges both when understanding others verbally and expressing themselves verbally and this limits their social relationships their readiness to learn new information and their adaptation to new environments (Edition, 2013). For example, visual aids are an adaptable and effective method for assisting individuals with disabilities in navigating, comprehending their physical and social surroundings, grasping abstract concepts, and articulating thoughts (Arthur-Kelly et al., 2009). Visual aids and AAC systems offer graphic visual stimuli to improve the understanding and learning of individuals with communication disabilities, notably among children with autism (Shane et al., 2009).

The potential for AR/VR to bridge the digital gap is enormous, as these technologies provide new avenues for online networking that are accessible to people with disabilities (Macdonald & Clayton, 2017; Watling, 2011). Immersive technology will advance into every life area including work and all aspects of communication through the introduction of the Metaverse's multi-user socially collaborative and pervasive principles (Parker et al., 2023). A recent study has investigated immersive technologies and virtual environments for individuals with various disabilities to demonstrate the possibilities of this developing technology (Kuhlen & Dohle, 1995). This has resulted in a variety of projects within fundamental areas, including assistive AR/VR hardware and software solutions. Significant contributions to innovative hardware infrastructures encompass assistive technologies for individuals with physical disabilities (Draganov & Boumbarov, 2015), non-invasive cognitive control apparatuses for gaming (Hawsawi & Semwal, 2014), and enhancements to user autonomy and management within smart home settings (Tang et al., 2015). Software-based AR/VR solutions have concentrated on several application domains (e.g., assistive visual systems Du and Bulusu 2021; Ruta et al., 2018 and supportive audio apps Mahmud et al., 2022), prioritizing the delivery of accessible user experiences.

The IoT enables AI to offer many promising solutions for making life simpler for disabled individuals. IoT connects devices through technology enabling new disruptive solutions to support impaired individuals while promoting inclusion of all (Alenizi & Al-Karawi, 2021). Internet of Things (IoT) enabled assistive devices and apps help disabled people gain independence along with better service access and improve their life quality (Vasco, 2020). The continuous surveillance and support of healthcare accessibility and mobility are regulated by technology devices under the IoT, which are equipped with connectivity, sensors, and actuators. Healthcare response times and treatment planning capabilities improve through wearable technology by tracking patient vital signs which doctors receive in real-time (Alenizi & Al-karawi, 2023). Smart home technology automates processes, enhancing accessibility and allowing individuals to manage their surroundings via voice commands or other adaptable interfaces (Almusaed et al., 2023). Further, navigation systems powered by the IoT improve accessibility and mobility in public areas, facilitating disabled individuals to move around buildings, streets, and public transportation.

The IoT, powered by AI, is a revolutionary technological shift that unites computing and communications. The internet reports from the intensive therapy unit (ITU) illustrate a society in which intelligent equipment is seamlessly interconnected and possesses digital identities (ID) (Lachtar et al., 2017). Through the use of internet connectivity and new technologies such as embedded sensors, real-time geolocation, and radio-frequency identification (RFID), commonplace items will soon be able to perceive, comprehend, and react to their surroundings (Amaral et al., 2011). This technical advancement enables the emergence of novel modes of interaction between individuals, the objects with which they interact, and the objects themselves (Tan & Wang, 2010). In general, AI could greatly benefit disabled individuals by easing the creation of interactive gadgets that increase physical accessibility and independence. This chapter delves into how AI is already making a positive impact in this field, and the way it possesses the capability to make future improvements to the lives of individuals with impairments.

7.2 AI Redefining Independence for the Disabled

7.2.1 Communication

A significant challenge encountered by individuals with disabilities is the ability to communicate effectively with others. Nonetheless, the capabilities of AI can enhance communication for individuals with diverse disabilities (Kumar et al., 2024). Computer programs powered by AI can help users visualize conversations by expressing themselves through text and graphics. Technology that can transform written information into spoken language is also helpful for people with neurological disorders or paralysis.

New opportunities for accessibility for people with impairments have emerged with the advent of AI voice-assisted systems like Alexa, Google Home, and Echo (Dieker et al., 2024). The use of AI makes it easier for people with disabilities to obtain information by allowing them to simply give orders to their gadgets. The reason behind this is the crucial role that AI plays in communication and engagement. People having trouble speaking can benefit from the development of speech-to-text and text-to-speech technology. Voice systems such as Voiceitt can adapt to the pronunciation of speakers over time, converting the user's spoken words into clear and standardized speech, which can be delivered as audio or text messages (Ahmad et al., 2025). The application can also assist individuals with speech impairments in facilitating face-to-face communication with one another. To help people with speech impairments communicate more effectively, Google developed Parrotron, an artificial intelligence tool that transforms their speech patterns into natural-sounding speech (Dutt et al., 2024). Google's Parrotron, also converts distorted speech into coherent dialogue, assisting individuals with speech impairments. Such developments also foster an inclusive workplace where people with disabilities can engage equally and collaboratively. AI is capable of monitoring communication tasks, thereby guaranteeing that disabilities do not impede participation. By identifying clients with impairments and tailoring customer service to their needs, AI can help firms increase satisfaction and loyalty.

Advances in artificial intelligence have made it possible to create assistive devices that improve the quality of life for individuals with hearing loss. "Google translator for the deaf and mute" (Mehta et al., 2023) is a common way to describe GnoSys, a well-known developer of AI-powered solutions. To translate hand motions or sign language into text and voice, the app makes use of AI, particularly computer vision and neural networks. A system that properly interprets whole words has been built by Google's DeepMind using AI-driven lip-reading algorithms (Mitra et al., 2023). After training on more than 5,000 h of TV shows, the system was able to decode 118,000 phrases. The research resulted in a system that can understand human speech in public settings, regardless of the level of background noise or lighting.

Artificial Intelligence has the potential to generate significant opportunities for visually impaired individuals. Technology for image recognition enables artificial intelligence to comprehend the context of objects within photographs and to provide descriptions of these images to individuals. Microsoft's Seeing AI serves as an exemplary computer vision platform that provides narration of the surrounding environment for visually impaired individuals by reading text, describing physical appearances, and recognizing faces and emotions (Lee et al., 2022). OrCam is a cutting-edge AI-powered gadget that enables the visually handicapped and blind to access live video feeds in response to voice instructions (Thakur et al., 2024). The device is capable of reading texts aloud from various sources, including books, newspapers, smartphone screens, and other printed or digital surfaces. Furthermore, it is capable of recognizing faces, as well as recognizing colors, items, and other visual components. It enables individuals with visual impairments to perform various tasks independently, enhancing their autonomy.

7.2.2 Educational Support

Everyone has a fundamental right to an education, and no one should be denied that right because of a disability. Despite the long history of assistive technologies like Braille and subtitles, AI is revolutionizing the way students learn. Artificial intelligence enables the customization of learning and training courses to address the unique requirements of each individual (Chen et al., 2020). Augmented and virtual reality technologies create interactive learning environments that are accessible to all students, regardless of ability, and promote diversity and tolerance in the classroom (Pramanik, 2024). This method guarantees that all individuals, irrespective of their capabilities, have the chance to acquire knowledge and develop. Ava is a communication application that utilizes artificial intelligence to assist individuals having hearing impairments (ElHennawy, 2024). It provides immediate transcriptions to facilitate group discussions and assists in the rapid composition of an initial draft. Everyone has the right to fully engage in a classroom discussion, including those suffering from hard of hearing.

7.2.3 Promoting an Independent Lifestyle

Solutions powered by artificial intelligence assist in establishing an autonomous personal and professional lifestyle for individuals with disabilities. A prevalent misunderstanding exists regarding individuals with disabilities, suggesting that they require constant assistance, which may lead to feelings of insecurity. Visually impaired people can use Envision AI to help them navigate interior and outdoor spaces. It offers comprehensive audio guidance for a more secure travel experience (Seiple et al., 2025). Additionally, blind people can use smart canes attached to smart glasses with having mic and speakers along with smart shoes for assisting in mobility (Fig. 7.1). For individuals who are physically disabled or paralyzed, one might assume that living independently is unattainable. Sesame Enable is one example of an artificial intelligence technology that enables users to improve their mobility and navigation by using facial motions (Xie et al., 2407). A virtual assistant, such as Google Assistant or Amazon's Alexa, can do a lot of things with simply voice commands, such as creating reminders and organizing meetings (Bogdan et al., 2021). Artificial intelligence allows people to focus on more meaningful activities by automating routine manual work. These innovations help remove social obstacles and open doors for disabled individual to live good self-sufficient lives.

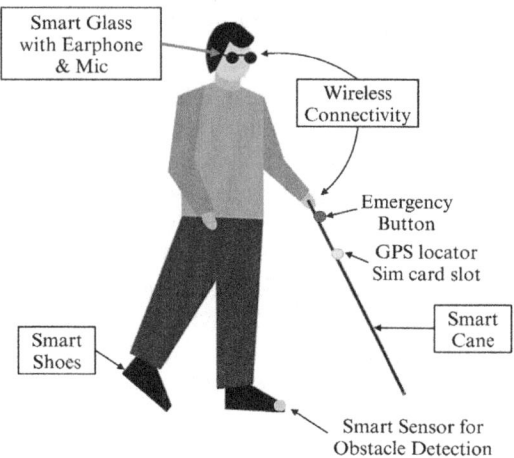

Fig. 7.1 Smart cane, smart glass, and smart shoes assisting in the mobility of blind individuals

7.2.4 Healthcare

The integration of AI in the medical sector possesses the potential to assist numerous individuals worldwide by facilitating faster and more precise diagnoses, which can result in more effective treatments, especially for those with disabilities. Several medical conditions can be better understood and treated with the help of AI systems, including cancer, rare diseases, high-risk pregnancies, and early detection of mental illnesses like schizophrenia and dementia (Brasil et al., 2019). In the context of disability support, AI allows healthcare personnel to focus on vital patient care by streamlining lesser activities. This leads to quicker identification of diseases, thereby decreasing the time and expenses usually involved in consulting multiple physicians. Artificial intelligence (AI) allows for less invasive surgical operations by coordinating machines to carry them out with less human intervention (Vitiello et al., 2012). Artificial intelligence enhances the diagnostic process; frequently, multiple hospital visits and significant financial resources are required solely for obtaining a diagnosis. The AI tools developed by Zebra Medical Vision allow for quicker and more precise diagnostics (Medida et al., 2025). Neuroprosthetics are a part of it; they help people with neurological deficits by enhancing the nervous system through electrical stimulation. The potential for AI to assume a variety of responsibilities is a frequently asked question. Better healthcare for all is a result of AI's practical improvements to medical workflows, clinical documentation, and patient outreach (Alowais et al., 2023).

7.2.5 Smart Homes Promoting Independent Living

The integration of AI into residential environments offers significant advantages for individuals with physical disabilities or mental health conditions. With the use of motion sensors, artificial intelligence can control various gadgets, allowing users to do things like turn on lights and fans just by lifting their hands or moving their heads (Fig. 7.2) (Siam et al., 2025). Sensors can identify unusual behavior in dementia patients and notify caregivers accordingly. Smart home technology offers significant advantages for individuals with limited mobility. Voice commands have made it possible for people to control nearly every aspect of their house with ease, from lighting to temperature to the stove to music playback, all with the simple expression of needs and requests (Ammari et al., 2019). With the help of smart home technology that is powered by AI, people with impairments may move around their homes more easily and lead more independent lives. Additionally, artificial intelligence aids elderly individuals or those with restricted mobility in performing tasks such as housekeeping, grooming, managing medications, eating, and carrying or transporting heavy objects (Nithikathkul et al., 2024).

Furthermore, software such as Mario Kompai, which aims to deliver genuine emotions and feelings, employs service robots to aid patients with mental health conditions, providing support and companionship (Whelan et al., 2020). For people with a variety of health issues, this technology greatly enhances the standard of living by allowing them to remain independent and safe in their own homes. Following that, Amazon Alexa is a great tool for people with disabilities since it allows them to talk

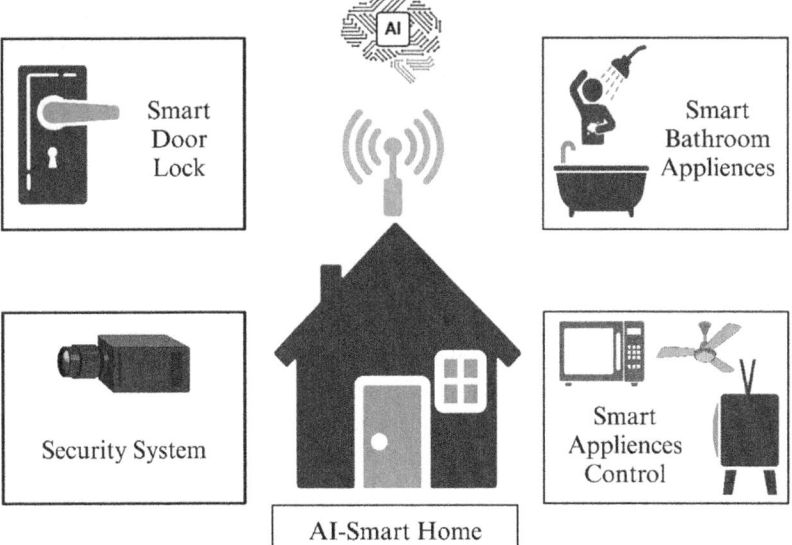

Fig. 7.2 AI-based smart home control devices

to the device, set alarms and reminders, listen to music, make to-do lists, and get up-to-the-minute information (Setiawan, 2024). People having trouble moving around may find the Smart Doorbell to be a very useful product. They can remotely access or unlock the door and see who's at the door through a monitoring screen. Disabled people's quality of life is improved by the accessibility and convenience offered by smart home equipment including smart lights, smart drapes, smart garage openers, and smart thermostats (Dini et al., 2024). Smart lighting can be utilized to remotely activate and deactivate lights, as well as to adjust the intensity of lighting within the home. Smart curtain technology enables the automatic opening and closing of curtains through a mobile application. Smart garage openers enable homeowners to oversee their garage door remotely using their smartphones. Smart thermostats are equipped with various features that enable users to adjust the home temperature remotely, ensuring comfort at all times (Tamas et al., 2024).

7.2.6 Increasing Accessibility

Persons with limited physical mobility may find their capabilities enhanced by artificial intelligence technologies. The goal of Microsoft's AI for Accessibility program is to promote social inclusion for people with disabilities by developing AI-powered solutions to the many cognitive and physical barriers that these people face in their daily lives and at work (Gupta & Khang, 2024). The goal of Microsoft's program is to help people with disabilities be more self-reliant and productive in their daily lives, at work, and in communication. For people with disabilities, that are typically housebound due to their condition, the advent of self-driving automobiles and other forms of autonomous transportation presents enormous mobility options. Companies like Google's Waymo, Lyft, Uber, and Drive AI have developed autonomous vehicles with the use of artificial intelligence. This could lead to people being less physically isolated and more likely to lead social lives (Ushakov et al., 2022). The utilization of driverless cars allows individuals with disabilities to access their homes, navigate their communities, engage with others, and seek employment opportunities. Autonomous vehicles could revolutionize mobility when fully integrated into society, making them more accessible and accommodating to different abilities and demands (Campisi et al., 2021).

AI-driven solutions can profoundly affect individuals with impairments by aiding them in daily tasks and promoting the development of new skills. Artificial intelligence technology aids individuals with impairments by establishing new pathways for accessibility, social inclusion, and independent living that may otherwise be difficult or unachievable (Setiawan, 2024). As AI advances, it possesses the capability to provide more sophisticated and innovative solutions for tackling the complex challenges encountered by individuals with disabilities, thereby promoting greater inclusion.

7.2.7 IOT for People with Disabilities

The Internet of Things (IoT) comprises a vast network of networked devices that collect data from the physical environment, offering several conveniences and improvements to daily life. While many studies have explored the general potential and privacy concerns of the IoT, there is a deficiency of research specifically addressing the privacy implications of IoT use by those with disabilities. More research on the specific requirements and preferences of people with disabilities is necessary because they constitute more than 15% of the world's population (Vasco, 2020). The development of Internet of Things (IoT) devices and services that are accessible to people with disabilities can improve their quality of life and open up new avenues for inclusion and accessibility (Abdelwahab et al., 2024). The IoT can transform the lives of those with disabilities by augmenting safety, mobility, and autonomy, thereby strengthening privacy. The IoT technology has spawned numerous new gadgets and services designed to fulfill the requirements of disabled individuals, to empower them, and diminish their dependence on external support. Accessibility and independence for people with disabilities have been greatly improved by assistive technologies that are AI-based and connected to the Internet of Things (Das et al., 2017). Adapting to the user's motions and providing real-time feedback, internet-connected prosthetics incorporating Internet of Things (IoT) sensors enhance mobility and usefulness. Individuals who are visually handicapped can benefit from smart shoes equipped with vibrating sensors and Internet of Things technology. These shoes provide directional cues for safe travel. Through voice commands or adaptive interfaces, users of Internet of Things (IoT) enabled smart home systems can manage temperature, lighting, and appliances to suit their individual needs. To provide prompt medical treatments and individualized care, wearable health monitors continuously record vital signs and health indices. People with speech impairments can communicate better, connect more effectively, and access vital services with the help of assistive communication devices that incorporate speech recognition technology and the Internet of Things.

These examples show the way AI-based IoT can enhance the lives of disabled people by giving them more independence, making their homes safer, and opening doors to more social opportunities. With the generation of IoT technology, there is a tremendous possibility for further game-changing applications in this field. While there are many benefits to accessible Internet of Things (IoT) devices and services, there are also some drawbacks, such as the potential for collecting more data on those with disabilities (Tsatsou, 2020). A major benefit of bridging the "data divide" is that it solves the problem of insufficient access to high-quality data on specific people or groups. Closing this gap could lead to better legislation, more efficient resource allocation, and the development of better products and services that are specifically designed to meet the requirements of those with disabilities. This might help reduce economic and social inequality in the long run (Hollier & Abou-Zahra, 2018).

In addition, for accessibility to be improved, designs must be universal and accessible. Universal design entails the development of products, structures, public areas, and activities that are accessible to the broadest spectrum of individuals. Conversely, accessible design prioritizes the explicit consideration of those with impairments in the design process. This plan ensures that all members of society, not only those with impairments, benefit from new Internet of Things technologies like closed-captioning and virtual assistants. It is worth mentioning that auto-complete and voice-recognition functions, which are today widely used, were initially created to assist individuals with disabilities in using computers (Rghioui & Oumnad, 2018). This idea, which has been called the "curb-cut effect" illustrates innovations that help persons with disabilities also benefit society as a whole. Originally designed for wheelchair users, curb cuts now accommodate a wide variety of pedestrians, including parents pushing strollers and individuals going grocery shopping. Ultimately, accessible Internet of Things devices have a multiplicity of positive impacts, including better quality of life, greater inclusion, and the lives of people with disabilities (Mouha, 2021).

7.3 Visual Supports as Visual Language

Researchers (Shane et al., 2014) developed a model for "visual language" that considers the prevalence of visual signals and assistive audiovisual devices. This model encompasses three modes: visual expressive (for expression), visual instructional (for comprehension), and visual organizational. In addition, studies have shown that visual learning modes are primarily supported by two types of traditional visual aids used in the classroom: visual activity schedules, which display a daily calendar or order of events for planning purposes, and structured visuals, which offer instructions for specific tasks as they are being carried out. Research on children at risk for emotional and behavioral disorders in preschool and primary school classrooms has shown that visual supports, when used in combination with instructional activities, social stories, and behavioral support interventions, boost student engagement and, more significantly, help students maintain consistency in their performance (Zimmerman et al., 2020).

On the other hand, users may become disengaged from their communication contexts due to a disconnect between the tools they use and their actual surroundings. Integrating visual aids and AAC systems in the future will require innovative and evolving technology. Considering the recent advancements in wristwatch and mobile device technologies, researchers (Schlosser et al., 2017) examined Apple WatchVR to find out if wearable devices could give "just-in-time" visual aids to children with intellectual disabilities and autism spectrum disorder (ASD) (Bryant & Hemsley, 2024; Schlosser et al., 2017). The researchers used a case study experimental design to see if providing visual aids helped participants successfully finish a tabletop activity. Both static and dynamic scene presentations appeared to benefit the children, and the Apple WatchVR was seen as an effective, undetectable, and unobtrusive way to offer visual aid.

7.3.1 Augmented Reality Delivering Visual Supports

One new technology that possesses the capability to enhance the engagement of communication aids with the environment is augmented reality (AR). Augmented reality allows users to enhance or modify their visual perception by superimposing computer-generated graphics onto their actual physical surroundings. These graphics may consist of holographic items, avatars, or instructional imagery, which includes textual text, graphics, or films (Carmigniani et al., 2011). A user creates an augmented environment by superimposing digital information on top of their real-world view using a camera-equipped mobile device or an augmented reality "glasses" system (like Google Glass or Microsoft HoloLens 2). An AR head-mounted display offers the advantage of hands-free observation of the enhanced environment. Anyone can participate and immerse themselves in their environment without needing a smart gadget. The wireless gadget is attached to an adjustable head strap. On the front there is a small computer that displays images on a see-through lens and on the back, there is a battery (Bryant & Hemsley, 2024).

7.3.2 Assistive AR/VR Developments

Numerous studies have shown that novel hardware systems and augmented/virtual reality software might be helpful for people with disabilities. Research has investigated applications for users with physical disabilities that support rehabilitation (Souza et al., 2019), physiotherapy (Basílio et al., 2018), biomechanical movement (Barioni et al., 2017), and the stabilization of involuntary physical motion, such as hand tremors (Wang et al., 2018). In addition, studies on immersive technology have looked at wheelchair-friendly interfaces and interactive gaming systems (Cuzzort & AstroWheelie, 2008). Research has demonstrated that immersive technologies can serve as visual assistance for people with visual impairments, enhancing contextual awareness and facilitating sensory substitution (Granquist et al., 2021). Additionally, research has concentrated on innovative interaction approaches to enhance users' spatial awareness (Coughlan & Miele, 2017) and on creating new user interaction strategies that integrate object localization with spatial audio (Katz et al., 2012) and echolocation (Andrade et al., 2021). To help people with visual impairments who use new interfaces for immersive technology, haptic interactions have been used to enable sensory substitution (Kim, 2020). Furthermore, studies have investigated the potential of feed-forward algorithms in immersive technologies to assist visually impaired individuals with virtual interactions (Lang & Machulla, 2021).

Researchers are investigating the innovative solutions that AR/VR may offer for individuals with neurodiversity and cognitive deficits, particularly in manipulating and targeting the sensory, interpersonal, motor, and cognitive processes that affect atypical developmental trajectories (Farroni et al., 2022). Numerous studies have examined the efficacy of immersive experiences as supplemental tools for people with various neurological disorders, such as dyslexia (Thelijjagoda et al., 2019), dysgraphia (Abid et al., 2019), and dyscalculia (Avila-Pesantez et al., 2018). Patients suffering from dementia, mild cognitive impairments (MCI), or age-related cognitive decline can now benefit from AR and VR therapy (Thapa et al., 2020). Assistance for individuals with autism spectrum disorder (ASD) (Zhao et al., 2021), attention deficit hyperactivity disorder (ADHD) (Alqithami et al., 2019), obsessive–compulsive disorder (OCD) (Cullen et al., 2021), and dyspraxia (difficulty with performing coordinated movements) (Dhanalakshmi et al., 2020) have dominated the study on intellectual and developmental disabilities.

The improvement of communication and social involvement for individuals who are Deaf and Hard of Hearing (DHH) has been the focus of research, with a focus on developing new accessible solutions (Izaguirre et al., 2020). Studies have focused on AR and VR systems which provide visual aids to enhance communication, such as speech bubble representations of dialogues (Peng et al., 2018) and the utilization of technologies like Automatic Speech Recognition (ASR) to improve visual aspects of social interactions (Mirzaei et al., 2012). Digital human representation and avatar cooperation (Waldow & Fuhrmann, 2020), interactive stories (Zainuddin et al., 2010), and instructional textbooks (Xu et al., 2020) are some of the ways that ASR has been used in AR/VR. Moreover, research has examined the extent to which augmented reality software might enhance social communication and the depiction of broader social environments, particularly in facilitating vocal pronunciation and language acquisition (Xu et al., 2020) as well as parent–child communication (Tenesaca et al., 2019). More recent research on augmented reality and virtual reality assistive software has revealed novel AR/VR tools for displaying sign language communication (Nazareth et al., 2014) and for easing the localization of objects in enhanced settings (Mirzaei et al., 2021).

7.4 AI-Driven Autonomous Cars for Disability Mobility

Walking speed and crossing decisions are among the most extensively investigated risk factors for pedestrians (Schwartz et al., 2022). Research indicates that the behaviors and choices of disabled pedestrians, rather than environmental or social factors, present the greatest risk. Investigations in these domains have resulted in an enhanced understanding of human movement and the design of environments that are both engaging and functional. The goal of the automobile industry's research and development efforts is to create cars with intelligence-enhancing technology, with the eventual goal of a completely autonomous vehicle. There are five tiers of vehicle automation according to groups like SAE and the National Highway Traffic Safety Administration (NHTSA). These levels progress from "full driver control" (i.e., no human intervention) to "full autonomous" (i.e., the vehicle handles all driving duties independently) (Park et al., 2018).

The objectives of autonomous vehicles include significantly decreasing traffic accidents, alleviating congestion, lowering pollution levels, and reducing transportation expenses. The social acceptability and integration of self-driving cars into the road traffic ecology will determine their eventual success or failure, regardless of the technical hurdles that still need to be overcome (Lahijanian & Kwiatkowska, 2016). Researchers identify reliability and trust as primary concerns for individuals utilizing self-driving cars. Reliability denotes a vehicle's capacity to handle unforeseen circumstances, whereas trust pertains to ensuring the safety of the vehicle. The substitution of human drivers with autonomous control systems may lead to significant challenges in social interaction (Rasouli & Tsotsos, 2019). To keep traffic flowing smoothly and safely, especially at pedestrian crossings, self-driving vehicles and pedestrians must communicate continuously. Together, autonomous vehicles and impaired pedestrians can do a lot of things, like recognize each other, anticipate where the pedestrians will go, assess their actions, exchange information, and obtain feedback from the vehicle (Kaur & Rampersad, 2018). The spread of agreements between pedestrians and automobiles through broadcasting techniques and edge computing is another objective of car-to-car communication tasks.

To drive safely in a congested environment, a self-driving car needs obstacle management capabilities. Accordingly, individual detection is an essential function for autonomous vehicles to drastically decrease the likelihood of accidents in the vehicular traffic system (Ragesh & Rajesh, 2019). The disabled represent a specific category of pedestrians navigating the road environment that have disabilities, including individuals who are blind, deaf, or use wheelchairs, among others. It is believed that self-driving cars will create numerous opportunities for individuals with disabilities, enhancing their independence and improving their quality of life. These vehicles will interact with users to facilitate greater mobility, autonomy, and confidence, particularly when navigating roadways (Reyes-Muñoz & Guerrero-Ibáñez, 2022). The ability to connect with automobiles and the mutual understanding of this contact is crucial for disabled pedestrians to feel safe in vehicular traffic environments (Imrie, 2012). So, to determine the way autonomous vehicles interact with pedestrians and with one another, a comprehensive communication system is required. It is critical that this framework can detect impairments, set up ways for people with disabilities to communicate with self-driving cars, and allow for wireless networking connections between vehicles.

Assistive technology (AT) has emerged as a result of recent efforts to enable these people through the use of technology. Any piece of hardware, piece of software, or piece of equipment that enhances the capabilities and features of people with impairments is considered assistive technology (AT) according to the Assistive Technology Industry Association (ATiA) (Guerrero-Ibañez et al., 2023). The World Health Organization indicates that assistive technology aims to empower individuals to live independently, maintain health, and engage productively, facilitating a more natural integration into society. Assistive technology can be utilized in various fields, including healthcare, education, and athletics.

7.4.1 Pedestrian-Autonomous Vehicle Interaction

An essential factor that influences the efficacy of autonomous cars is their capacity to engage with pedestrians. Research on enhancing the interaction between autonomous cars and pedestrians has shown minimal advancement. Serious consequences might result from inadequate pedestrian-vehicle communication (Merat et al., 2018). For instance, consider a scenario in which the vehicle is aware of the intentions of the pedestrians. In that scenario, the vehicle is capable of responding and preventing a collision with the pedestrian, thereby mitigating the risk of significant harm to the pedestrian, which may include fatal consequences. The lack of a driver in an autonomous vehicle generates ambiguity among pedestrians over the actions of the self-driving car (Reig et al., 2018).

The majority of interaction initiatives have concentrated on transmitting messages from autonomous vehicles to pedestrians. These notifications provide pedestrians with the essential instructions to take the appropriate action. Visual, auditory, and anthropomorphic interfaces are the three main categories into which the developed interaction technologies fall (Löcken et al., 2019). Some studies have suggested visual interfaces, which may include things like projections or holograms, screens that display text or icons, or LED strips (Deb et al. 2018; Habibovic et al., 2018). This activity is intended to be communicated to the pedestrian by each of these user interfaces. To improve message transmission for the visually impaired, researchers are investigating ways to complement visual interfaces with auditory devices (Lee et al., 2021). Anthropomorphic interfaces are designed to communicate essential tasks to pedestrians by utilizing human characteristics, such as the ability to mimic the appearance of eyes to establish eye contact (Ochiai & Toyoshima, 2011).

Nevertheless, further advancements are required in establishing a method for pedestrians to interact with autonomous vehicles. A major concern will be the vehicle's comprehension of pedestrians' intentions. For effective communication between a pedestrian and a self-driving automobile, the vehicle must be trained to accurately interpret the pedestrian's signals. Numerous studies examine posture (Fang & López, 2019; Le et al., 2022; Mínguez et al., 2018), head position (Perdana et al., 2021; Rehder et al., 2014), and the trajectory and kinematics of pedestrians (Huang et al., 2020; Quan et al., 2021). The primary issue with these methods was their dependence on implicit communication. The autonomous vehicle deduces the pedestrian's intentions from their activities in this kind of communication. One study explored the potential for autonomous vehicles and pedestrians to communicate directly using basic hardware devices that utilize IEEE 802.11p wireless technology. Following this, the autonomous car discreetly notifies nearby autonomous vehicles with pedestrian alerts and information, and it also takes into account hand signals to indicate that the pedestrian wants to use the intersection.

7.4.2 Key Factors in Pedestrian-Autonomous Vehicle Communication

Pedestrians and autonomous vehicles need to be able to communicate with each other in a way that is both easy and secure. This requires a system that is both flexible and easy to understand. According to the researchers (Mahadevan et al., 2018), there are two crucial steps that the autonomous car must take to engage with the pedestrian. The primary focus of the first stage is for the self-driving car to locate and recognize any pedestrians in its path. The second level indicates that autonomous vehicles must inform pedestrians of their intended actions. By the stages detailed by the researchers (Mahadevan et al., 2018), supplementary steps will be required for the specific interaction process between automated self-driving vehicles and disabled individuals.

7.4.3 Pedestrian Detection

Detecting all objects or impediments inside the vehicle's travel surroundings is necessary for the autonomous navigation functions of ASCs. Object detection enables the autonomous vehicle to compute its trajectory or determine the necessary action to avert situations that could jeopardize the safety of others around. Finding objects, measuring their distance and location, and keeping a comprehensive record of all things (static and dynamic) are the key functions of the ASC. However, owing to the enormous processing needs for large data sets, object recognition and classification pose substantial hurdles. Therefore, such function is handled by technologies that use machine learning and deep learning. The two primary approaches to object identification and classification in ASCs are feature extraction and object classification. By segmenting and reducing raw input into smaller, more manageable groupings for processing, feature extraction involves data dimensionality reduction. Forms, angles, and motion can be better identified in digital images and videos using this method. The Histogram of Oriented Gradients (Zhang et al., 2020), the Deformable Part Model (Li et al., 2018), the Local Binary Pattern (Kaur & Nazir, 2021), and the Aggregate Channel Feature (ACF) (Huang et al., 2021) are among the present feature extraction approaches.

Disabled people can be located and classified using a variety of DL methodologies. Some deep learning models, such CNNs, can achieve classification rates of one hundred percent or more (Li et al., 2018). After defining possible areas or locations where the item might be present, the region-based method employs a convolutional neural network (CNN) model to generate a detection box. Regional Convolutional Neural Networks (R-CNNs) (Chen et al., 2018; Shi et al., 2018), Mask Region-based CNNs (Malbog, 2019; Shen et al., 2020), and Fast and Faster R-CNNs (Zhao et al., 2021; Zhu et al., 2019) are all examples of such network architectures. Additionally, the concept of regions is not employed by regression-based algorithms. Regression of the category and target boundary across several image points is made possible by processing the input image a single time. You Only Look Once (YOLO) (Redmon et al., 2016), Single-Shot MultiBox Detector (SSD) (Liu et al., 2016), and RetinaNet (Ross & Dollár, 2017) are all algorithms that fall into this category. YOLO is a popular model for real-time object detection; it can process video at 30 frames per second, which is faster than other models, but it lacks detection accuracy.

7.5 Conclusion

The incorporation of artificial intelligence has significantly influenced life, especially for those with impairments. Prominent corporations such as Google, Microsoft, and Apple persist in advancing breakthrough AI-driven solutions, fostering a more inclusive and diverse society in which all individuals are afforded equal chances. Artificial intelligence technologies are transforming disability assistance by streamlining both routine and intricate tasks, dismantling obstacles, and promoting enhanced autonomy. Through breakthroughs in communication, education, and healthcare, AI is improving accessibility and empowerment for those with disabilities. Furthermore, AI-enhanced smart homes, IoT integration, and advanced AR/VR technologies are revolutionizing the interaction of individuals with impairments with their environment. The future of AI has potential for autonomous cars, enhancing mobility and autonomy. As technology advances, AI will persist in transforming independence, fostering a more inclusive, accessible, and equitable environment for individuals with disabilities. The continuous progress in AI-driven support indicates a future in which technology closes divides and promotes equitable involvement in society.

References

Abdelwahab, M. M., Al-Karawi, K. A., Hasanin, E. M., & Semary, H. E. (2024). Autism spectrum disorder prediction in children using machine learning. *Journal of Disability Research, 3*(1), 20230064.

Abid, M., Bhimra, M. A., Mubeen, M., Zahid, A. B., & Shahid, S. (2019, June 12). Peppy: A paper-based augmented reality application to help children against dysgraphia. In *Proceedings of the 18th ACM International Conference on Interaction Design and Children* (pp. 544–549).

Ahmad, W., Shokeen, R., & Raj, R. (2025). Artificial intelligence: Solutions in special education. In *Transforming special education through artificial intelligence* (pp. 459–520). IGI Global.

Alenizi, A. S., & Al-Karawi, K. A. (2022). Cloud computing adoption-based digital open government services: Challenges and barriers. In *Proceedings of Sixth International Congress on Information and Communication Technology: ICICT 2021, London* (Vol. 3, pp. 149–160). Springer.

Alenizi, A. S., & Al-karawi, K. A. (2023, February 20). Machine learning approach for diabetes prediction. In *International Congress on Information and Communication Technology* (pp. 745–756). Springer Nature Singapore.

References

Almusaed, A., Yitmen, I., & Almssad, A. (2023). Enhancing smart home design with AI models: A case study of living spaces implementation review. *Energies, 16*(6), 2636.

Alowais, S. A., Alghamdi, S. S., Alsuhebany, N., Alqahtani, T., Alshaya, A. I., Almohareb, S. N., Aldairem, A., Alrashed, M., Bin Saleh, K., Badreldin, H. A., & Al Yami, M. S. (2023). Revolutionizing healthcare: The role of artificial intelligence in clinical practice. *BMC Medical Education, 23*(1), 689.

Alqithami, S., Alzahrani, M., Alzahrani, A., & Mostafa, A. (2019). Modeling an augmented reality game environment to enhance behavior of adhd patients. In *Brain Informatics: 12th International Conference, BI 2019, Haikou, China, December 13–15, 2019, Proceedings 12 2019* (pp. 179–188). Springer International Publishing.

Amaral, L. A., Hessel, F. P., Bezerra, E. A., Corrêa, J. C., Longhi, O. B., & Dias, T. F. (2011). ECloudRFID–A mobile software framework architecture for pervasive RFID-based applications. *Journal of Network and Computer Applications, 34*(3), 972–979.

Ammari, T., Kaye, J., Tsai, J. Y., & Bentley, F. (2019). Music, search, and IoT: How people (really) use voice assistants. *ACM Transactions on Computer-Human Interaction (TOCHI), 26*(3), 1–28.

Andrade, R., Waycott, J., Baker, S., & Vetere, F. (2021). Echolocation as a means for people with visual impairment (PVI) to acquire spatial knowledge of virtual space. *ACM Transactions on Accessible Computing (TACCESS), 14*(1), 1–25.

Arthur-Kelly, M., Sigafoos, J., Green, V., Mathisen, B., & Arthur-Kelly, R. (2009). Issues in the use of visual supports to promote communication in individuals with autism spectrum disorder. *Disability and Rehabilitation, 31*(18), 1474–1486.

Avila-Pesantez, D. F., Vaca-Cardenas, L. A., Delgadillo Avila, R., Padilla Padilla, N., & Rivera, L. A. (2018, August 29). Design of an augmented reality serious game for children with dyscalculia: a case study. In *International Conference on Technology Trends* (pp. 165–175). Springer International Publishing.

Barioni, R. R., Chaves, T. M., Figueiredo, L., Teichrieb, V., Neto, E. V., & Da Gama, A. E. (2017, November 1). Arkanoidar: An augmented reality system to guide biomechanical movements at sagittal plane. In *2017 19th Symposium on Virtual and Augmented Reality (SVR)* (pp. 207–214). IEEE.

Basílio, S. D., Ferreira, A. L., do Nascimento, D. G., & Silva, R. S. (2018, October 28). Augmented reality as mirror therapy in post stroke treatment. In *2018 20th Symposium on Virtual and Augmented Reality (SVR)* (pp. 220–224). IEEE.

Bogdan, R., Tatu, A., Crisan-Vida, M. M., Popa, M., & Stoicu-Tivadar, L. (2021). A practical experience on the Amazon Alexa integration in smart offices. *Sensors, 21*(3), 734.

Brasil, S., Pascoal, C., Francisco, R., dos Reis Ferreira, V. A., Videira, P., & Valadão, G. (2019). Artificial intelligence (AI) in rare diseases: Is the future brighter? *Genes, 10*(12), 978.

Bryant, L., & Hemsley, B. (2024). Augmented reality: A view to future visual supports for people with disability. *Disability and Rehabilitation: Assistive Technology, 19*(3), 800–813.

Campisi, T., Severino, A., Al-Rashid, M. A., & Pau, G. (2021). The development of the smart cities in the connected and autonomous vehicles (CAVs) era: From mobility patterns to scaling in cities. *Infrastructures, 6*(7), 100.

Carmigniani, J., Furht, B., Anisetti, M., Ceravolo, P., Damiani, E., & Ivkovic, M. (2011). Augmented reality technologies, systems and applications. *Multimedia Tools and Applications, 51*, 341–377.

Chen, E., Tang, X., & Fu, B. (2018, July 16). A modified pedestrian retrieval method based on faster R-CNN with integration of pedestrian detection and re-identification. In *2018 International Conference on Audio, Language and Image Processing (ICALIP)* (pp. 63–66). IEEE.

Chen, L., Chen, P., & Lin, Z. (2020). Artificial intelligence in education: A review. *IEEE Access, 8*, 75264–75278.

Coughlan, J. M., & Miele, J. (2017, October 9). AR4VI: AR as an accessibility tool for people with visual impairments. In *2017 IEEE International Symposium on Mixed and Augmented Reality (ISMAR-Adjunct)* (pp. 288–292). IEEE.

Cullen, A. J., Dowling, N. L., Segrave, R., Carter, A., & Yücel, M. (2021). Exposure therapy in a virtual environment: Validation in obsessive compulsive disorder. *Journal of Anxiety Disorders, 80*, 102404.

Cuzzort, S., & Starner, T. (2008, September 28). AstroWheelie: A wheelchair based exercise game. In *2008 12th IEEE International Symposium on Wearable Computers* (pp. 113–114). IEEE.

Das, R., Tuna, A., Demirel, S., & Yurdakul, M. K. (2017). A survey on the internet of things solutions for the elderly and disabled: Applications, prospects, and challenges. *International Journal of Computer Networks and Applications, 4*(3), 1–9.

Deb, S., Strawderman, L. J., & Carruth, D. W. (2018). Investigating pedestrian suggestions for external features on fully autonomous vehicles: A virtual reality experiment. *Transportation Research Part f: Traffic Psychology and Behaviour, 59*, 135–149.

de Souza, R. F., Farias, D. L., da Rosa, R. C., Damasceno, E. F. (2019 October 28). Analysis of low-cost virtual and augmented reality technology in case of motor rehabilitation. In *2019 21st Symposium on Virtual and Augmented Reality (SVR)* (pp. 161–164). IEEE.

Dhanalakshmi, B., Dhanagopal, R., Raguraman, D., & Thamdapani, T. (2020, December 3). Improving cognitive learning of children with dyspraxia using selection based mid-air gestures in athynos game. In *2020 3rd International Conference on Intelligent Sustainable Systems (ICISS)* (pp. 231–237). IEEE.

Dieker, L., & Zaugg, T. (2024, April 9). Artificial intelligence and the intersectionality of disability. In *The Palgrave encyclopedia of disability* (pp. 1–8). Springer Nature Switzerland.

Dini, P., Paolini, D., Saponara, S., & Minossi, M. (2024). Leaveraging digital twin & artificial intelligence in consumption forecasting system for sustainable luxury yacht. *IEEE Access*.

Draganov, I. R., & Boumbarov, O. L. (2015, September 24). Investigating Oculus Rift virtual reality display applicability to medical assistive system for motor disabled patients. In *2015 IEEE 8th International Conference on Intelligent Data Acquisition and Advanced Computing Systems: Technology and Applications (IDAACS)* (Vol. 2, pp. 751–754). IEEE.

Du, P., & Bulusu, N. (2021, October 17). An automated AR-based annotation tool for indoor navigation for visually impaired people. In *Proceedings of the 23rd International ACM SIGACCESS Conference on Computers and Accessibility* (pp. 1–4).

Dutt, S., Kanauzia, R., & Bartwal, H. (2024). Multilayer perceptron-based speech emotion recognition for identifying the problematic skills of dyslexic learners. In *Artificial intelligence and machine learning* 2024 (pp. 113–124). CRC Press.

Edition, F. (2013). Diagnostic and statistical manual of mental disorders. *American Psychiatric Association, 21*(21), 591–643.

ElHennawy, S. M. (2024). The impact of Artificial Intelligence (AI) in the assessment and treatment of communication disorders (a review of literature). *The Egyptian Journal of Language Engineering, 11*(2), 36–45.

Fang, Z., & López, A. M. (2019). Intention recognition of pedestrians and cyclists by 2d pose estimation. *IEEE Transactions on Intelligent Transportation Systems, 21*(11), 4773–4783.

Farroni, T., Valori, I., & Carnevali, L. (2022). Multimedia interventions for neurodiversity: Leveraging insights from developmental cognitive neuroscience to build an innovative practice. *Brain Sciences, 12*(2), 147.

Granquist, C., Sun, S. Y., Montezuma, S. R., Tran, T. M., Gage, R., & Legge, G. E. (2021). Evaluation and comparison of artificial intelligence vision aids: Orcam myeye 1 and seeing ai. *Journal of Visual Impairment & Blindness, 115*(4), 277–285.

Guerrero-Ibañez, J., Contreras-Castillo, J., Amezcua-Valdovinos, I., & Reyes-Muñoz, A. (2023). Assistive self-driving car networks to provide safe road ecosystems for disabled road users. *Machines, 11*(10), 967.

Gupta, C., & Khang, A. (2024). Designing artificial intelligence-enabled training approaches and models for physical disabilities individuals. In *AI-oriented competency framework for talent management in the digital economy* (pp. 388–415). CRC Press.

References

Habibovic, A., Lundgren, V. M., Andersson, J., Klingegård, M., Lagström, T., Sirkka, A., Fagerlönn, J., Edgren, C., Fredriksson, R., Krupenia, S., & Saluäär, D. (2018). Communicating intent of automated vehicles to pedestrians. *Frontiers in Psychology, 9*, 1336.

Hawsawi, O., & Semwal, S. K. (2014, October 5). EEG headset supporting mobility impaired gamers with game accessibility. In *2014 IEEE International Conference on Systems, Man, and Cybernetics (SMC)* (pp. 837–841). IEEE.

Hollier, S., & Abou-Zahra, S. (2018, April 23). Internet of things (IoT) as assistive technology: Potential applications in tertiary education. In *Proceedings of the 15th International Web for All Conference* (pp. 1–4).

Huang, K., Li, J., Liu, Y., Chang, L., & Zhou, J. (2021, October 6). A survey on feature point extraction techniques. In *2021 18th International SoC Design Conference (ISOCC)* (pp. 201–202). IEEE.

Huang, Z., Hasan, A., Shin, K., Li, R., & Driggs-Campbell, K. (2020). Long-term pedestrian trajectory prediction using mutable intention filter and warp LSTM. *IEEE Robotics and Automation Letters, 6*(2), 542–549.

Imrie, R. (2012). Auto-disabilities: The case of shared space environments. *Environment and Planning A, 44*(9), 2260–2277.

Izaguirre, E. D., Abásolo, M. J., & Collazos, C. A. (2020, October 19). Mobile technology and extended reality for deaf people: A systematic review of the open access literature. In *2020 XV Conferencia Latinoamericana de Tecnologías de Aprendizaje (LACLO)* (pp. 1–8). IEEE.

Katz, B. F., Kammoun, S., Parseihian, G., Gutierrez, O., Brilhault, A., Auvray, M., Truillet, P., Denis, M., Thorpe, S., & Jouffrais, C. (2012). NAVIG: Augmented reality guidance system for the visually impaired: Combining object localization, GNSS, and spatial audio. *Virtual Reality, 16*, 253–269.

Kaur, N., & Nazir, N. (2021, September 3). A review of local binary pattern based texture feature extraction. In *2021 9th International Conference on Reliability, Infocom Technologies and Optimization (Trends and Future Directions) (ICRITO)* (pp. 1–4). IEEE.

Kaur, K., & Rampersad, G. (2018). Trust in driverless cars: Investigating key factors influencing the adoption of driverless cars. *Journal of Engineering and Technology Management, 48*, 87–96.

Kim, J. (2020). VIVR: Presence of immersive interaction for visual impairment virtual reality. *IEEE Access, 8*, 196151–196159.

Kuhlen, T., & Dohle, C. (1995). Virtual reality for physically disabled people. *Computers in Biology and Medicine, 25*(2), 205–211.

Kumar, V., Barik, S., Aggarwal, S., Kumar, D., & Raj, V. (2024). The use of artificial intelligence for persons with disability: A bright and promising future ahead. *Disability and Rehabilitation: Assistive Technology, 19*(6), 2415–2417.

Lachtar, A., Kachouri, A., & Val, T. (2017, February 17). Real-time monitoring of elderly using their connected walking stick. In *2017 International Conference on Smart, Monitored and Controlled Cities (SM2C)* (pp. 48–52). IEEE.

Lahijanian, M., & Kwiatkowska, M. (2016, September 28). Social trust: A major challenge for the future of autonomous systems. In *2016 AAAI Fall Symposium Series*.

Lang, F., & Machulla, T. (2021, December 8). Pressing a button you cannot see: Evaluating visual designs to assist persons with low vision through augmented reality. In *Proceedings of the 27th ACM Symposium on Virtual Reality Software and Technology* (pp. 1–10).

Le, M. C., Do, T. D., Duong, M. T., Nguyen, V. B., & Le, M. H. (2022, August 17). Skeleton-based recognition of pedestrian crossing intention using attention graph neural networks. In *2022 International Workshop on Intelligent Systems (IWIS)* (pp. 1–5). IEEE.

Lee, J., Park, W., & Lee, S. (2021, June 28). Discovering the design challenges of autonomous vehicles through exploring scenarios via an immersive design workshop. In *Proceedings of the 2021 ACM Designing Interactive Systems Conference* (pp. 322–338).

Lee, S., Yu, R., Xie, J., Billah, S. M., & Carroll, J. M. (2022, March 22). Opportunities for human-AI collaboration in remote sighted assistance. In *Proceedings of the 27th International Conference on Intelligent User Interfaces* (pp. 63–78).

Li, J., Wong, H. C., Lo, S. L., & Xin, Y. (2018). Multiple object detection by a deformable part-based model and an R-CNN. *IEEE Signal Processing Letters, 25*(2), 288–292.

Li, Y., Cui, F., Xue, X., & Chan, J. C. (2018). Coarse-to-fine salient object detection based on deep convolutional neural networks. *Signal Processing: Image Communication, 64*, 21–32.

Light, J., McNaughton, D., & Caron, J. (2019). New and emerging AAC technology supports for children with complex communication needs and their communication partners: State of the science and future research directions. *Augmentative and Alternative Communication, 35*(1), 26–41.

Liu, W., Anguelov, D., Erhan, D., Szegedy, C., Reed, S., Fu, C. Y., & Berg, A. C. (2016). SSD: Single shot multibox detector. In *Computer Vision–ECCV 2016: 14th European Conference, Amsterdam, The Netherlands, October 11–14, 2016, Proceedings, Part I 14 2016* (pp. 21–37). Springer International Publishing.

Löcken, A., Golling, C., & Riener, A. (2019, September 21). How should automated vehicles interact with pedestrians? A comparative analysis of interaction concepts in virtual reality. In *Proceedings of the 11th International Conference on Automotive User Interfaces and Interactive Vehicular Applications* (pp. 262–274).

Macdonald, S. J., & Clayton, J. (2017, October 2). Back to the future, disability and the digital divide. In *Disability and technology* (pp. 128–144). Routledge.

Mahadevan, K., Somanath, S., & Sharlin, E. (2018, April 21). Communicating awareness and intent in autonomous vehicle-pedestrian interaction. In *Proceedings of the 2018 CHI Conference on Human Factors in Computing Systems* (pp. 1–12).

Mahmud, M. R., Stewart, M., Cordova, A., & Quarles, J. (2022, March 12). Auditory feedback for standing balance improvement in virtual reality. In *2022 IEEE Conference on Virtual Reality and 3D User Interfaces (VR)* (pp. 782–791). IEEE.

Malbog, M. A. (2019, December 20). MASK R-CNN for pedestrian crosswalk detection and instance segmentation. In *2019 IEEE 6th International Conference on Engineering Technologies and Applied Sciences (ICETAS)* (pp. 1–5). IEEE.

Medida, L. H., Kumar, G. L., & Prasad, M.(2025). Transformative AIoT applications in medicine: Real-world case studies. In Future innovations in the convergence of AI and internet of things in medicine (pp. 367–406). IGI Global Scientific Publishing.

Mehta, P., Chillarge, G. R., Sapkal, S. D., Shinde, G. R., & Kshirsagar, P. S. (2023). Inclusion of children with special needs in the educational system, Artificial Intelligence (AI). In *AI-assisted special education for students with exceptional needs* (pp. 156–185). IGI Global.

Merat, N., Louw, T., Madigan, R., Wilbrink, M., & Schieben, A. (2018). What externally presented information do VRUs require when interacting with fully automated road transport systems in shared space? *Accident Analysis & Prevention, 118*, 244–252.

Mínguez, R. Q., Alonso, I. P., Fernández-Llorca, D., & Sotelo, M. A. (2018). Pedestrian path, pose, and intention prediction through gaussian process dynamical models and pedestrian activity recognition. *IEEE Transactions on Intelligent Transportation Systems, 20*(5), 1803–1814.

Mirzaei, M. R., Ghorshi, S., & Mortazavi, M. (2012, May 28). Combining augmented reality and speech technologies to help deaf and hard of hearing people. In *2012 14th Symposium on Virtual and Augmented Reality* (pp. 174–181). IEEE.

Mirzaei, M., Kán, P., & Kaufmann, H. (2021, March 27). Multi-modal spatial object localization in virtual reality for deaf and hard-of-hearing people. In *2021 IEEE Virtual Reality and 3D User Interfaces (VR)* (pp. 588–596). IEEE.

Mitra, S., Lakshmi, D., & Govindaraj, V. (2023). Data analysis and machine learning in AI-assisted special education for students with exceptional needs. In *AI-assisted special education for students with exceptional needs* (pp. 67–109). IGI Global.

Mouha, R. A. (2021). Internet of things (IoT). *Journal of Data Analysis and Information Processing, 9*(2), 77.

Nazareth, D. R., Alencar, M. A., & Netto, J. F. (2014, May 12). Elra-teaching brazilian sign language using augmented reality. In *2014 XVI Symposium on Virtual and Augmented Reality* (pp. 110–113). IEEE.

References

Nithikathkul, C., Meenorngwar, C., Krates, J., & Kijphati, R. (2024). Mobile application for improving the quality of life and elderly health care. *International Journal of Geoinformatics, 20*(7), 100–117.

Ochiai, Y., & Toyoshima, K. (2011, March 13). Homunculus: The vehicle as augmented clothes. In *Proceedings of the 2nd Augmented Human International Conference* (pp. 1–4).

Olszewski, P., Szagała, P., Rabczenko, D., & Zielińska, A. (2019). Investigating safety of vulnerable road users in selected EU countries. *Journal of Safety Research, 68*, 49–57.

Park, H., Khattak, Z., & Smith, B. (2018, March). Glossary of connected and automated vehicle terms. *Connected Vehicle Pool Fund Study*.

Parker, C., Yoo, S., Lee, Y., Fredericks, J., Dey, A., Cho, Y., & Billinghurst, M. (2023, April 19). Towards an inclusive and accessible metaverse. In *Extended Abstracts of the 2023 CHI Conference on Human Factors in Computing Systems* (pp. 1–5).

Peng, Y. H., His, M. W., Taele, P., Lin, T. Y., Lai, P. E., Hsu, L., Chen, T. C., Wu, T. Y., Chen, Y. A., Tang, H. H., & Chen, M. Y. (2018, April 21) Speechbubbles: Enhancing captioning experiences for deaf and hard-of-hearing people in group conversations. In *Proceedings of the 2018 CHI Conference on Human Factors in Computing Systems* (pp. 1–10).

Perdana, M. I., Anggraeni, W., Sidharta, H. A., Yuniarno, E. M., & Purnomo, M. H. (2021, July 21). Early warning pedestrian crossing intention from its head gesture using head pose estimation. In *2021 International Seminar on Intelligent Technology and Its Applications (ISITIA)* (pp. 402–407). IEEE.

Pramanik, S. (2024). Immersive innovations: Exploring the use of virtual and augmented reality in educational institutions. In *Augmented reality and the future of education technology* (pp. 66–85). IGI Global.

Quan, R., Zhu, L., Wu, Y., & Yang, Y. (2021). Holistic LSTM for pedestrian trajectory prediction. *IEEE Transactions on Image Processing, 30*, 3229–3239.

Ragesh, N. K., & Rajesh, R. (2019). Pedestrian detection in automotive safety: Understanding state-of-the-art. *IEEE Access, 7*, 47864–47890.

Rasouli, A., & Tsotsos, J. K. (2019). Autonomous vehicles that interact with pedestrians: A survey of theory and practice. *IEEE Transactions on Intelligent Transportation Systems, 21*(3), 900–918.

Redmon, J., Divvala, S., Girshick, R., & Farhadi, A. (2016). You only look once: Unified, real-time object detection. In *Proceedings of the IEEE Conference on Computer Vision and Pattern Recognition* (pp. 779–788).

Rehder, E., Kloeden, H., & Stiller, C. (2014, October 8). Head detection and orientation estimation for pedestrian safety. In *17th International IEEE Conference on Intelligent Transportation Systems (ITSC)* (pp. 2292–2297). IEEE.

Reig, S., Norman, S., Morales, C. G., Das, S., Steinfeld, A., & Forlizzi, J. (2018, September 23). A field study of pedestrians and autonomous vehicles. In *Proceedings of the 10th International Conference on Automotive User Interfaces and Interactive Vehicular Applications* (pp. 198–209).

Reyes-Muñoz, A., & Guerrero-Ibáñez, J. (2022). Vulnerable road users and connected autonomous vehicles interaction: A survey. *Sensors, 22*(12), 4614.

Rghioui, A., & Oumnad, A. (2018). Challenges and opportunities of internet of things in healthcare. *International Journal of Electrical & Computer Engineering (2088-8708), 8*(5).

Ross, T. Y., & Dollár, G. K. (2017, July). Focal loss for dense object detection. In *Proceedings of the IEEE Conference on Computer Vision and Pattern Recognition* (pp. 2980–2988).

Ruta, D., Jordan, L., Fox, T. J., Boakes, R. (2018, April 23). WebSight: Using AR and WebGL shaders to assist the visually impaired. In *Proceedings of the 15th International Web for All Conference* (pp. 1–2).

Schlosser, R. W., O'Brien, A., Yu, C., Abramson, J., Allen, A. A., Flynn, S., & Shane, H. C. (2017). Repurposing everyday technologies to provide just-in-time visual supports to children with intellectual disability and autism: A pilot feasibility study with the Apple Watch®. *International Journal of Developmental Disabilities, 63*(4), 221–227.

Schreibman, L., Dawson, G., Stahmer, A. C., Landa, R., Rogers, S. J., McGee, G. G., Kasari, C., Ingersoll, B., Kaiser, A. P., Bruinsma, Y., & McNerney, E. (2015). Naturalistic developmental behavioral interventions: Empirically validated treatments for autism spectrum disorder. *Journal of Autism and Developmental Disorders, 45*, 2411–2428.

Schwartz, N., Buliung, R., Daniel, A., & Rothman, L. (2022). Disability and pedestrian road traffic injury: A scoping review. *Health & Place, 77*, 102896.

Seiple, W., van der Aa, H. P., Garcia-Piña, F., Greco, I., Roberts, C., & van Nispen, R. (2025). Performance on activities of daily living and user experience when using artificial intelligence by individuals with vision impairment. *Translational Vision Science & Technology, 14*(1), 3.

Semary, H. E., Al-Karawi, K. A., Abdelwahab, M. M., & Elshabrawy, A. M. (2024). A Review on Internet of Things (IoT)-related disabilities and their implications. *Journal of Disability Research, 3*(2), 20240012.

Setiawan, A. (2024, November 15). Intelligent systems for disabilities technology for a more inclusive life. Available at SSRN 5062273.

Shane, H. C., Laubscher, E., Schlosser, R. W., Fadie, H. L., Sorce, J. F., Abramson, J. S., Flynn, S., & Corley, K. (2014). Enhancing communication for individuals with autism: A guide to the visual immersion system. *Brookes*.

Shane, H. C., O'Brien, M., & Sorce, J. (2009). Use of a visual graphic language system to support communication for persons on the autism spectrum. *Perspectives on Augmentative and Alternative Communication, 18*(4), 130–136.

Shen, G., Jamshidi, F., Dong, D., & ZhG, R. (2020, September 12). Metro pedestrian detection based on mask R-CNN and spatial-temporal feature. In *2020 IEEE 3rd International Conference on Information Communication and Signal Processing (ICICSP)* (pp. 173–178). IEEE.

Shi, P., Wu, J., Wang, K., Zhang, Y., Wang, J., & Yi, J. (2018, November 7). Research on low-resolution pedestrian detection algorithms based on R-CNN with targeted pooling and proposal. In *2018 Eighth International Conference on Image Processing Theory, Tools and Applications (IPTA)* (pp. 1–5). IEEE.

Siam, S. I., Ahn, H., Liu, L., Alam, S., Shen, H., Cao, Z., Shroff, N., Krishnamachari, B., Srivastava, M., & Zhang, M. (2025). Artificial intelligence of things: A survey. *ACM Transactions on Sensor Networks, 21*(1), 1–75.

Tamas, R., O'Brien, W., & Agee, P. (2024). Thermostat standardization, technology trends, future considerations: Expert interviews. *Energy and Buildings, 325*, 114946.

Tan, L., & Wang, N. (2010, August 20). Future internet: The internet of things. In *2010 3rd International Conference on Advanced Computer Theory and Engineering (ICACTE)* (Vol. 5, pp. V5–376). IEEE.

Tang, L. Z., Ang, K. S., Amirul, M., Yusoff, M. B., Tng, C. K., Alyas, M. D., Lim, J. G., Kyaw, P. K., & Folianto, F. (2015, April 7). Augmented reality control home (ARCH) for disabled and elderlies. In *2015 IEEE Tenth International Conference on Intelligent Sensors, Sensor Networks and Information Processing (ISSNIP)* (pp. 1–2). IEEE.

Tenesaca, A., Oh, J. Y., Lee, C., Hu, W., & Bai, Z. (2019, October 10). Augmenting communication between hearing parents and deaf children. In *2019 IEEE International Symposium on Mixed and Augmented Reality Adjunct (ISMAR-Adjunct)* (pp. 431–434). IEEE.

Thakur, R., Thakur, A., Viral, R., & Asija, D. (2024, June 21). AI based visual impairment system for blind and people with least reading capabilities. In *2024 IEEE Students Conference on Engineering and Systems (SCES)* (pp. 1–5). IEEE.

Thapa, N., Park, H. J., Yang, J. G., Son, H., Jang, M., Lee, J., Kang, S. W., Park, K. W., & Park, H. (2020). The effect of a virtual reality-based intervention program on cognition in older adults with mild cognitive impairment: A randomized control trial. *Journal of Clinical Medicine, 9*(5), 1283.

Thelijjagoda, S., Chandrasiri, M., Hewathudalla, D., Ranasinghe, P., & Wickramanayake, I. (2019, August 19). The hope: An interactive mobile solution to overcome the writing, reading and speaking weaknesses of dyslexia. In *2019 14th International Conference on Computer Science & Education (ICCSE)* (pp. 808–813). IEEE.

Tsatsou, P. (2020). Digital inclusion of people with disabilities: A qualitative study of intra-disability diversity in the digital realm. *Behaviour & Information Technology, 39*(9), 995–1010.

Ushakov, D., Dudukalov, E., Shmatko, L., & Shatila, K. (2022). Artificial Intelligence as a factor of public transportations system development. *Transportation Research Procedia, 63*, 2401–2408.

Vasco, L. N. (2020). Internet of Things feasibility for disabled people. *Transactions on Emerging Telecommunications Technologies, 31*(12), e3906.

Vitiello, V., Lee, S. L., Cundy, T. P., & Yang, G. Z. (2012). Emerging robotic platforms for minimally invasive surgery. *IEEE Reviews in Biomedical Engineering, 6*, 111–126.

Waldow, K., & Fuhrmann, A. (2020, March 22). Addressing deaf or hard-of-hearing people in avatar-based mixed reality collaboration systems. In *2020 IEEE Conference on Virtual Reality and 3D User Interfaces Abstracts and Workshops (VRW)* (pp. 594–595). IEEE.

Wang, K., Matsukura, H., Iwai, D., & Sato, K. (2018). Stabilizing graphically extended hand for hand tremors. *IEEE Access, 6*, 28838–28847.

Watling, S. (2011). Digital exclusion: Coming out from behind closed doors. *Disability & Society, 26*(4), 491–495.

Whelan, S., Burke, M., Barrett, E., Mannion, A., Kovačič, T., Santorelli, A., Luz Oliveira, B., Gannon, L., Shiel, E., & Casey, D. (2020). The effects of MARIO, a social robot, on the resilience of people with dementia: A multiple case study. *Gerontechnology*.

World Health Organization. (2018). World Health Organization Road Traffic Injuries. Erişim Adresi: https://www.who.int/news-room/fact-sheets/detail/road-traffic-injuries (Erişim Tarihi: 14.07. 2019).

Xie, J., Yu, R., Zhang, H., Lee, S., Billah, S. M., & Carroll, J. M. (2024, July 11). Emerging practices for large multimodal model (lmm) assistance for people with visual impairments: Implications for design. arXiv:2407.08882.

Xu, D., Ma, Z., Jian, Z., Shi, L., Wang, L., & Gao, J. (2020, November 13). Speech rehabilitation system for hearing impaired children based on virtual reality technology. In *2020 International Conference on Virtual Reality and Visualization (ICVRV)* (pp. 209–212). IEEE.

Zainuddin, N. M., Zaman, H. B., & Ahmad, A. (2010, May 7). A participatory design in developing prototype an augmented reality book for deaf students. In *2010 Second International Conference on Computer Research and Development* (pp. 400–404). IEEE.

Zhang, L., Zhou, W., Li, J., Li, J., & Lou, X. (2020, December 8). Histogram of oriented gradients feature extraction without normalization. In *2020 IEEE Asia Pacific Conference on Circuits and Systems (APCCAS)* (pp. 252–255). IEEE.

Zhao, Z., Ma, J., Ma, C., & Wang, Y. (2021, November 19). An improved faster R-CNN algorithm for pedestrian detection. In *2021 11th International Conference on Information Technology in Medicine and Education (ITME)* (pp. 76–80). IEEE.

Zhao, J. Q., Zhang, X. X., Wang, C. H., & Yang, J. (2021). Effect of cognitive training based on virtual reality on the children with autism spectrum disorder. *Current Research in Behavioral Sciences, 2*, 100013.

Zhu, K., Li, L., Hu, D., Chen, D., & Liu, L. (2019, December 11). An improved detection method for multi-scale and dense pedestrians based on Faster R-CNN. In *2019 IEEE International Conference on Signal, Information and Data Processing (ICSIDP)* (pp. 1–5). IEEE.

Zimmerman, K. N., Ledford, J. R., Gagnon, K. L., & Martin, J. L. (2020). Social stories and visual supports interventions for students at risk for emotional and behavioral disorders. *Behavioral Disorders, 45*(4), 207–223.

The manufacturer's authorised representative in the EU is Springer Nature Customer Service Centre GmbH, Europaplatz 3, 69115 Heidelberg, Germany. If you have any concerns regarding our products, please contact ProductSafety@springernature.com

Printed and bound by CPI Group (UK) Ltd, Croydon, CR0 4YY

27/03/2026

02080143-0004